Nine-Day Inner Cleansing and Blood Wash for Renewed Youthfulness and Health

by

I. E. GAUMONT
Therapeutic Researcher

in association with

HAROLD E. BUTTRAM, M.D.

REWARD BOOKS

Library of Congress Cataloging-in-Publication Data

Gaumont, I. E.
  Nine-day inner cleansing and blood wash for renewed
youthfulness and health.
      p. cm.
  Includes index.
  ISBN 0-13-622506-3
  1. Diet therapy.   2. Nutrition.   3. Reducing diets.
  4. Rejuvenation.   I. Buttram, Harold E.
  joint author.   II. Title.
  RM216.G275   1980   79-19590
  616.2   CIP

Printed in the United States of America

40   39

This book is a reference work based on research by the author. The opinions expressed herein are not necessarily those of or endorsed by the publisher. The directions stated in this book are in no way to be considered as a substitute for consultation with a duly licensed doctor.

ISBN 0-13-622506-3

ATTENTION: CORPORATIONS AND SCHOOLS

Prentice Hall books are available at quantity discounts with bulk purchase for educational, business, or sales promotional use. For information, please write to: Prentice Hall Special Sales, 240 Frisch Court, Paramus, New Jersey 07652. Please supply: title of book, ISBN number, quantity, how the book will be used, date needed.

Reward Books
Paramus, NJ 07652

On the World Wide Web at http://www.phdirect.com

Foreword

Very few people today would question the fact that we are living in an era of unparalleled pollution involving every phase of the human environment. In addition to air and water pollution, there are literally thousands of synthetic chemicals being added to commercial food products—chemicals which are almost all foreign to the biological systems of life. The foods themselves are seldom left in their life and health building states; they are adulterated, denatured, and devitalized by various forms of processing. In a manner of speaking, it would not be to too far amiss to say that we are living in an era of unprecedented blood pollution.

At this time, few would venture to predict the long range effects of this pollution on human biology and genetics, but we do know that there is a very real and significant statistical increase in various metabolic and degenerative diseases. There also appears to be an increasing number of people who are not suffering from any specific disease, but whose energies and vitality are at such low levels that they are able to meet the

minimal demands of daily routine only with the greatest difficulty. Any physician working in some phase of primary care for
the general public has a significant portion of patients whose
main complaints are those of extreme, persistent fatigue and
exhaustion accompanied by varying degrees of nervousness, irritability, and depression. Perhaps saddest of all are those who
have lost all capacity for enjoyment. For those a beautiful
sunset has no meaning. The fresh air of the woods brings no
exhilaration. There may even be a temporary loss of the
capacity for feeling warmth and affection for friends and family. Although causes are many and varied—and often not
directly the fault of the patient— it is basically true that
spiritual and mental health (as well as physical health) are impossible in a grossly polluted body.

On first reading *Nine-Day Inner Cleansing and Blood
Wash for Renewed Youthfulness and Health,* I was impressed
that Mr. I. E. Gaumont has prepared an unusually well
organized and comprehensive guide-book for those seeking
that rare and most cherished state of being known as *good
health.* At a time when there is already a large literature on this
topic, I believe that this book is a distinct contribution because
of its simplicity and workability. Also, it penetrates to the most
basic keys which are essential for those desiring health and a
higher fulfillment in their lives. It does this with an insight
which can only come from experience.

It must be admitted that many of the procedures outlined
here are based more on tradition than on the so-called scientific
method. This can scarcely be otherwise when one considers
that the health field, as a science, is in its infancy. It may require years or decades to gain scientific confirmation for some
of these methods which have come down to us from earlier
pioneers as a result of their observation, intuition, and genius.
In the meantime, on the basis of simple observation and experi-

ence, we know that these things work and that many are able to find their way back to health and to a more satisfying and enjoyable life as a result of their application.

Harold E. Buttram, M.D.

Medical Director Clymer Memorial Building
Medical Advisor Clymer Health Center, Quakertown, Pennsylvania

Memberships in the:

American College of Applied Nutrition
American Academy of Preventive Medicine
American Academy of Medical Preventics

A Word from the Author

I have written this book to reveal what I discovered to be the prime cause of disease, and to present my way of preventing and overcoming disease by natural means. The practical information in this book is the result of forty years of intensive study and therapeutic research. This information enables me to combat illness without the use of drugs.

Today, in spite of advances in medicine and the number of drugs now available, more people are sick, or devitalized, than ever before in the history of our country. Heart attacks are more prevalent than ever. There are approximately thirteen million people afflicted with the degenerative disease of arthritis. The crippling illness, diabetes, is taking its toll of millions.

You don't have to be sick anymore. I have discovered that a healthy body will overcome most diseases and common ailments with its own powers, if it is allowed to function properly. In many people, faulty eating habits and poor foods block body functions. If you eat intelligently, get enough rest, and avoid excessive stresses and strains, you body will fight off most diseases. Only after your body's defenses have been overcome will most diseases have a chance to grow within you.

There is a way to free your body of accumulated poisons that make you sick. I will show you how to cleanse yourself internally. Once you have done this, if you keep yourself internally clean, you can live to a ripe old age. I myself am enjoying life at the age of 83, and you can do the same. Mother Nature has planned that you live to be 100 years old; it is only internal problems in your system that might prevent this.

Anyone whose ill health is due to dietary errors is fortunate—especially when he or she discovers the truth early—because then the trouble can be easily remedied. Recent discoveries of science can bring you gratifying relief from aches and pains and a complete recovery from any illness in the offing. These discoveries relate to your internal conditions, the food you eat, and the food you should eat.

The freeing of your body from poisonous wastes which I describe in my Nine-Day Inner Cleansing and Blood Wash is accomplished through the healing power in certain foods. You know that proper diet is of more importance than any other factor in maintaining health. Without food, no life is possible. Without correct food, no health is possible.

Do not misunderstand me. Whenever I use the word "diet" in this book I do not mean merely a decrease in eating for the purpose of losing excess weight. In this book, diet describes a way to control eating for general health improvement. It may—and generally does—signify a change in the quality of food you eat as well as in its quantity. Such control results in loss of excess weight, but gives you many other benefits as well.

The Nine-Day Inner Cleansing and Blood Wash can bring about dramatic changes, and the general change in eating habits that follows it is a powerful weapon against disease, so miraculous it almost defies belief. This is a "breakthrough" of vital, world-wide importance.

The Nine-Day Inner Cleansing and Blood Wash for Renewed Youthfulness and Health will conquer disease in almost all cases by unlocking the natural powers of the body. This effective home treatment has accomplished this for me, for members of my family, and for many of my other relatives and friends.

It is hoped that there will be an increasing number of people, whether healthy or not, who will find that it is to their advantage to make use of this book for renewed youthfulness and health. Just reading it will make you feel better.

I. E. Gaumont

A Tribute to Harold E. Buttram, M.D.

It shows considerable broad-mindedness and courage for Harold E. Buttram, a doctor of medicine with orthodox qualifications, to expound the rationale of what many of his less broad-minded colleagues might well dismiss as nothing but "old wives' tales." When doctors express themselves in print, it is usually to draw learned attention to some new drug—and not to the remedial natural treatment of disease.

Dr. Buttram's endeavors are in the area of natural healing, with his medical methodology being used only to sustain the patient until the natural methods can correct the cause. Therefore, "all honor to Dr. Buttram."

The Author

Acknowledgments

I am deeply indebted to the late Helen Houston, world renowned nutritionist, teacher, and health lecturer, for her invaluable teachings on how to strike back at disease without the use of drugs.

The health-minded public at large would have sustained an irreparable loss had it not been for her ideals, her indomitable teachings of how to enjoy good life throughout life—and for her remarkable introduction of the principles leading to the Nine-Day Inner Cleansing and Blood Wash for Renewed Youthfulness and Health. Therefore, all honor to the late Helen Houston.

I am also grateful to Robin Clyde, news correspondent and columnist, for her scholarly editorial assistance in preparing the first draft of this book. I wish to pay special tribute to my wife, Connie, for her inspiration, encouragement, and invaluable contribution to the writing of this book.

About nature
Consult Nature herself

Lord Bacon

A little knowledge of health
is a dangerous thing.

The Author

Contents

Growth • A "Miracle" Recovery from Two Strokes • Cases of
Sinus Trouble Yield to Molasses-Therapy • Beneficial in
Menopause • Healthy and Easy Pregnancy • Overcoming
Anemia • Beneficial in Varicose Veins • Overcoming Erysipelas •
Speedy Recovery from Cancer of the Knee • A Case History of My
Own • Don't Make the Same Mistake I Made • The Most
Convenient Way of Taking Molasses • Cider Vinegar: A Wonder
Beverage • The Safest Cure for Obesity • Why a Common Table
Fluid Is So Beneficial • Modifying the Desire to Over-Eat • How
She Lost Her "Stenographer's Seat" • How She Improved Her
Heart Condition • How to Reduce Hemophilia to a Minimum •
How to Put a Stop to Frequent Nose-Bleeding • How to Cure a
Sore Throat Rapidly • How You Can Recover from a Tickling
Cough • How You Can Recover from Laryngitis in 7 Hours •
Helpful in a Mild Type of Asthma • How You May Restore Your
Mental and Physical Vigor • How You May Overcome
Heartburn and Digestive Trouble • How to Relieve Yourself of
Frequent Nicturation • Honey: A Food for Healing • Rich in
Vitamins and Minerals • How to Rid Your Body of Deadly Germs
• Overcoming Gastric Ulcers • The Valuable Elements in Honey
• Garlic: The Three-Thousand-Year-Old Miracle Medicine •
Avail Yourself of the Remarkable Restorative Powers of Garlic •
Spain's Mortality Rate Is Low Compared to the U.S. • How Mr.
C Recovered from Dangerously High Blood Pressure • How Miss
M Recovered from Mild Diabetes • How a Patient Recovered
from Diarrhea and High Blood Pressure • How Mrs. R's Little
Daughter Recovered from Sinus Problems

Dissipating the Possibility of Cancer of the Rectum •
Elimination of Digested Food Before Putrefaction Sets In •
Bowel Flushing Enemas Pay Off in Dividends • A Case History
Worthy of Note • A Way to Overcome Habitual Use of Harmful
Drug Laxatives • Outmoding Purgative Medicine • I Hold the
Key to a Locked Bowel • How to Overcome Obesity and Live
Longer • Why Overweight People Are Prone to Heart Disease •
Diet Pills Have "Extremely Limited" Value in Weight Loss
Programs • What to Do for "Quick Weight Loss" • Method • A
Pleasurable Way of Fasting • Could You Ask for Anything More?

Any Diet, Designed to Reduce Cholesterol Levels • Little-Known Health Ideas

Processed Foods, Synthetic Drugs and Chemicals in Vogue Today • Unprecedented Blood Pollution • 80 to 90% of Cancer Environmentally Caused • Eminent Religious Devotees Are Pioneers of Nutrition •Astounding Health of the Hunzas • Raw vs. Cooked • Relationship Between Sugar and Alcoholism • Mental Illness Brought About by Sugar Intake • Loss of Memory and Coordination from Chemical Food Additives • The Bill of Rights • The Concept of Blood Pollution • Individual Responsibility Concerning Matters of Health • We Are Living in a "Synthetic" Period • Why Our System Is Disease and Drug Oriented

Why the Body Must Be Healed and Not the Disease • Nature's Law of Compensation Against Every Disease • Why Deep Breathing Is Vital • The Beginning of Disease • How Right Living Brings Health • A Warning to Clean Up • "Ye Suffer from Yourselves; None Other Binds You That You Bloat and Die" • Disease: The Cure Is the Opposite of the Cause • A New Way of Fasting • A New Outlook on Life • God Doesn't Dwell in an Unclean Temple • The Body Is Yours to Mold • Foods and Their Chemical Elements

A Startling Secret Discovery • A Difficult Task in Store • Is a Change of Climate the Answer to Hay Fever? • Ragweed Pollen Takes Over • Not My Cup of Tea • Warm, Dry Climate the Best by Far • How and When I Contracted Hay Fever • A Step in the Right Direction • An Encouraging Discovery • Increasing the Dosage of Vitamin C • A Suggestion for My Hay Fever • Abstinence from Faulty Foods • The Happy Hour • Overcoming Allergic Ailments • Chronic Fatigue • Gastritis • High Blood Pressure • How to Slim Down Without Dieting or the Use of Drugs • Bronchitis • Sinusitis • A Home Remedy for Postnasal Drip • Acidosis • Shortness of Breath • Backache • Obesity

1

Conquering Disease with a Nine-Day Inner Cleansing and Blood Wash

Many illnesses can be conquered, and your health can improve tremendously if you give yourself an inner cleansing and blood wash. As you know, the cells of your body are nourished and cared for by your blood. To more fully understand the functions of your body, bear in mind that all life begins with the individual cell. Inside your body, it is an aggregation of closely interrelated cells, serving a common purpose, that makes up your individual tissues and organs. And it is the interrelationship of all of your organs and tissues that makes up your body.

While you usually think of your body as a unit, it is in reality a composite of billions of minute cells, each cell an independent unit of living matter. Each cell has a function interrelated with others, but it also possesses its own individual needs and requirements. Nutrition and drainage of each cell is carried on by your blood, and these functions are of paramount importance to the health of that cell.

Cell Stagnation

When your blood is not properly purified, stagnation takes place within your cells. There are many factors that lead to a stagnant cellular condition. One such factor is fatigue. Fatigue depletes your nervous energy and leads to an impairment of glandular secretions.

Another factor is overeating. When you overindulge in food, you contribute in a large measure to the stagnation of your cells. Overeating contributes to sluggish elimination of waste from cells, seriously interfering with the work of your cells and body organs and preventing the normal nutrition and drainage of cells by your blood.

In my opinion, a stagnant cellular condition in any human body—a condition involving all the billions of live cells in that body—makes it extremely difficult to isolate and eliminate any cells that are impaired. Thus, cell stagnation can contribute to cancerous conditions, especially breast cancer.

Many illnesses seem to be connected with cell stagnation. If your nose is "stuffed up" or congested, or if you experience congestion in your throat or chest, it indicates that there is an accumulation of stagnant matter within you. A catarrhal condition in any part of your body, expressed in the form of sinus trouble, bronchitis, asthma, or colitis, is the result of stagnation. Arthritis is an outgrowth of toxins that have accumulated in the body. Skin eruptions such as acne, eczema, hives, or pimples indicate an impairment of drainage and deficient nutrition.

Displaced body organs, loss of muscular tone, and general feelings of illness or debility are all due to a weakening of the tissues that results from retention of poisons related to poor blood circulation and sluggish elimination.

These conditions are the warnings that both the nutrition and the drainage of cells have become impaired and destruction within the cells is gaining the upper hand. Unless corrected, this will lead to premature aging and a decline in vigor and body function.

All this can be prevented by first giving the body an opportunity to cleanse and purify itself, and then rebuilding the body and its cells with proper foods.

Cell Rejuvenation

The purpose of the rejuvenating Nine-Day Inner Cleansing and Blood Wash is two-fold: first, to cause the greatest possible elimination of accumulated waste and toxins; and, secondly, to supply your body with live natural foods rich in minerals and vitamins in order to restore the elements needed for cell rejuvenation.

In this book, I am going to tell you exactly how to carry out this amazing self-treatment. I will describe how you can cleanse your inner system and purify your blood simply by eliminating certain foods and adding others to what you eat during a nine-day period.

The Nine-Day Inner Cleansing and Blood Wash is accomplished with sensible nutrition. When I first discovered for myself how vital nutrition was, only a few medical doctors admitted its importance, and they were among the most radical in their profession. But even then, thirty years ago, I predicted that the time would come when the study of foods and their relation to disease would become a respected part of medical study. That time is now here.

Today, a course in nutrition is considered a primary subject in medical schools and other institutions that teach the diagnosis and therapy of human disorders. I feel a certain amount of satisfaction in knowing that the most orthodox doctors are expounding that theory today.

Nutrition needs no apologies for its claim to importance
in the health field. Scientists have thoroughly investigated
the nutritional values, or lack of any, in foods. Teachings
about worthwhile foods and "junk" foods are founded upon
solid, irrefutable facts. Today, new discoveries about foods
and their functions within the body permit us to evaluate
foods even more thoroughly. When I first began my own
investigations, these matters were not so well known. I soon
discovered, however, that it is possible for a nutritional deficiency to be at the bottom of any disease, and that it is quite
possible for stored-up poisonous wastes in the human body to
contribute mightily to the effects of a disease.

My investigations had a very personal interest for me. In
my earlier years I was in a state of broken health. I suffered
from bronchitis, shortness of breath, sinusitis, gastritis,
acidosis, high blood pressure, constipation, chronic fatigue,
backache, obesity, and hay fever. This last condition had
plagued me for 20 years, and the doctors I consulted
concurred that it was incurable.

I noticed that doctors, as a rule, try to find cures but
seldom think of spending any time in seeking causes. This
gave me food for thought. I was struck with the idea that in
order to heal disease one should know what actually causes
disease. In quest of such knowledge, I spent considerable time
delving into old and new medical books and medical journals.
No one knew how to solve my problem, or was able to help.

Healing the Body First
When Illness Strikes

Then, when least expected, *Eureka*! The answer came. I
happened to attend one of the nightly classes conducted by
the late Helen Houston, world renowned nutritionist, health
lecturer, and teacher. Her subject was inner cleansing of the

body. She recommended very strongly that you "heal the body first" if you are afflicted with disease.

Heal the body first! I was startled to hear this. It struck a responsive chord in me. Her approach sounded perfectly rational and certainly worth a try. Helen Houston explained that disease in general is primarily an outgrowth of poisonous wastes, or toxins, that have accumulated and formed a lining around the intestinal wall in the human body from the time of childhood, blocking up the system with uneliminated and unnatural food substances built up over the years. She said that retention of such toxins clearly results in an impairment of body drainage, indicating that destruction in the body is gaining an upper hand, and unless corrected, it will further aggravate the conditions of persons suffering from disease.

I lost no time in employing the nine-day cleansing regimen she advised, and six months after completing it, repeated it for another nine day period. In the interim, I recast my eating habits, refraining from eating "wrong" foods and partaking of good, nutritional foods.

A Small Miracle

About a year later, a small miracle took me by extreme surprise. I found that I had recovered completely from my hay fever, and from all my allergic ailments. This was no surprise to Helen Houston, who matter-of-factly said that I was just another fortunate class member who was healed by inner cleansing. I venture to say that I found her regimen "tried and true."

Since that time I have continued to develop her inner cleansing teachings into my Nine-Day Inner Cleansing and Blood Wash. Again and again I have observed that one who is clean inside experiences renewed youthfulness and greater protection against common ailments.

A Secret Discovery
Revealed

I feel it is my duty as a humanitarian to pass on my life changing discovery of the Nine-Day Inner Cleansing and Blood Wash for Renewed Youthfulness and Health to those unfortunate people suffering from disease, and to those who are desirous of preventing disease before it strikes. An ounce of prevention is worth a pound of cure.

A *giant* of health, it will rid your body of poisonous wastes (toxins) that have accumulated and formed a lining around the intestinal wall since childhood—causing disease.

It will dissipate the possibility of cancer of the rectum, which is increasing at an astonishing rate.

It is a positive way to avoid ever having a heart attack.

It will reduce your weight without dieting or the use of drugs—and keep you slim during your lifetime.

The basic secret and central message is that you treat the cause of disease first and the symptoms second. When illness strikes, you "heal the body first," contrary to the approach of the many medical doctors who are irrationally and illogically extreme in their practice of attacking the disease first. Fortunately, however, there are many doctors today who have the courage of their convictions and are blazing new trails, so to speak.

Dr. Buttram is to be commended for daring to venture into unorthodox therapies. At his Clymer Health Complex, his main endeavors are in the area of natural healing, with medical methodology being used only to sustain the patient until the natural methods can correct the cause. His natural methods include traditional drugless healing systems plus many unique therapies and nutritional therapy.

Patients who have recovered completely from illnesses after employing the Nine-Day Inner Cleansing and Blood Wash swear by it.

No more dangerous drugs . . . . No more costly medical treatments.

It will reverse the aging process, and increase your longevity by 20 years.

Today, at the young age of 84 "going on 60," I am a well preserved individual, hale and hearty, mind as sharp as a razor and productively abundant. My weight has been reduced from 195 to 145 (give or take a little), and my waist from 44 to 34 inches. I am erect in stature, athletically inclined, with a full crop of silver-white hair and no wrinkles on my face.

My wife, Connie, at the young age of 70 "going on 50," hasn't been to a medical doctor in about 20 years.

I did not have occasion to see a doctor for a great number of years, until I reached the age of 65 when I thought it best to have periodical check-ups by a doctor of medicine. Old age symptoms are bound to crop up no matter how healthy you may be.

I suddenly developed a thyroid condition about three years ago. This can become serious in so many ways if allowed to remain. I recovered from it completely in thirty days—largely due to living a clean and healthful life.

When you reach the age of 65, see a doctor at least three times a year, even if it is just for checking your blood pressure.

The Nine-Day Inner Cleansing and Blood Wash has cured me of hay fever which plagued me for 20 summers . . . along with other allergic ailments.

- It may keep you alive if you have had a heart attack or stroke.
- It will heal arthritis if not in the advanced stages.
- It will lessen the intake of insulin by diabetics.
- It will obviate the occurrence of breast cancers, intestinal cancers, and cancerous growths in the body.

- It will restore your masculine vigor and put pow-wow in your sex life.
- It will overcome low blood sugar.
- It will aid in normalizing high blood sugar.
- It will overcome post nasal drip.
- It will overcome an urge to urinate too frequently.

Here are some case histories of people who were restored to health after employing the Nine-Day Inner Cleansing and Blood Wash for Renewed Youthfulness and Health:

David J., high school principal, recovered from constipation, high blood pressure, obesity, and sluggishness. His weight was reduced from 230 to 180 pounds.

Mary C., past middle age, spinster, teacher, and lecturer, recovered from persistent constipation and indigestion and a weight problem. She got welcome relief from chest, arm and leg pains caused by an accidental fall.

Mabel K. recovered from persistent palpitation of the heart, backache, shingles (herpes), and buzzing in her ears when she was trying to fall asleep at night. Her weight is down to 125, and her waist measurment is 25 inches. She is 57 years old.

Louis H., age 63, produce dealer and meat cutter, recovered from sinusitis, acidosis, post nasal drip, backache, leg pains, and high blood sugar.

Monte J., age 52, bachelor and inventor of toys, recovered from persistent high blood pressure, backache, leg pains, and obesity. His weight is down from 185 to 160 pounds.

Connie Gaumont, my wife, and a former ballerina, is 71 going on 50 and doesn't look a day older. She has not been to a medical doctor in over 20 years, not even for a check-up. She swears by the Nine-Day Inner Cleansing and Blood Wash for Renewed Youthfulness and Health.

What Happens During the Nine Days of Cleansing

During the nine "cleansing days," you will be restoring yourself by eliminating certain troublesome foods from your meals. You will be enjoying the clean, fresh taste of certain fruits and vegetables, preferably uncooked. If you are troubled with conditions such as colitis, gastritis, ulcers, and constipation, you can carry out the nine-day cleansing with cooked vegetables and fruits.

You can best treat yourself with the nine-day cleansing in late spring, when there is an abundance of seasonal fresh fruits and vegetables, but you make undertake it any time. For the first four days, you will continue eating these fruits and vegetables.

On the fifth day, you will begin the action which will effect a good, thorough wash of your bloodstream. You'll simply begin to sip certain fresh fruit juices. As I'll explain, the kind and quality of these juices is of great importance to the success of the blood wash.

On the sixth and seventh days you'll be eating an abundance of green salads and green vegetable juices—the greener the better—to supply you with the cleansing and purifying power of chlorophyll.

On the eighth and ninth days, you'll be drinking delicious fruit juices once again, to complete the restorative nature of this treatment.

Most people experience no difficulty during this nine-day period, but I'll explain just what do to if at any time you should feel even the slightest bit weak or dizzy.

My method requires that you drink fruit and vegetable juices, or eat fruits and vegetables, at different times. Since fruits and vegetables, as well as their respective juices, are digested in your body by separate enzyme systems, you will be able to digest and absorb them better when you do not take them at the same time.

What You Will Eat

I have chosen the following fresh fruits and vegetables to be eaten during your inner cleansing and blood wash because they are high in vitamins and minerals, and because they are greatly effective in the healing of disease.

You should clean your fruits and vegetables in water containing chlorine in sufficient quantity to have a definite bactericidal effect. (Do *not* add chlorine to the water, as too much can be harmful. Ordinary tap water contains a small quantity of chlorine.) Wash the fruits and vegetables thoroughly so as to render harmless any dangerous sprays which are used during the growing period.

CRANBERRY contains natural citric, malic and benzoic acids, acting as intestinal antiseptics and facilitating digestion. It is helpful in obesity, poor complexion, liver disorders, pimples, diarrhea, asthma, catarrh, and goitre.

APPLES are perhaps the most health-giving fruits that exist. "An apple a day keeps the doctor away" is no empty slogan, for apples contain some important chemical ingredients. They favor oxidation of the blood, tend to prevent intestinal putrefaction, regulate calcium metabolism, retard the onset of old age, and render the urine normal.

A Blood Builder

GRAPES assist the body in burning some of its stored fat, at the same time keeping the sugar from falling too low. As a good blood and body builder, they are helpful in liver disorders, anemia, jaundice, pimples, and skin diseases. They stimulate circulation, act as a mild laxative, and are also helpful in nervousness, reducing diets, and low blood pressure. They are not recommended for diabetics, or someone who is prone to diarrhea and hyperacidity.

Rich in Minerals

CELERY was used by Hippocrates, Greek philosopher and Father of Medicine, in the 5th Century, B.C. It is a mild diuretic and laxative, and it stimulates circulation. Every part of the plant is considered by nutritionists to be a beneficial food. The celery leaves are a good source of calcium and a high source of sodium, chlorine, and chlorophyll. Celery stalks are high in potassium. Here we find rich sources of vitamins A and B, and a wealth of minerals.

Celery is very helpful in arthritis, gout, sciatica, high blood pressure, rheumatism, obesity, insomnia, urinary disorders, chronic appendicitis, hyperacidity, headaches, neuritis, neuralgia, indigestion, cystitis, and dropsy. It is a good body and vitality builder.

Rich in Vitamins

LETTUCE is a good source of the four major vitamins, A, E, C and B. It is helpful in urinary disorders, insomnia, acidosis, obesity, catarrh, anemia, dyspepsia, and goitre, and it stimulates circulation. It is a good diuretic and laxative.

Helpful in
High Blood Pressure

PEARS contain small amounts of citric and malic acids. They are helpful in indigestion, high blood pressure, colitis, catarrh, and skin eruptions, and they tend to decrease the acidity of urine. Pears are *not recommended for diabetics.*

Helpful in
Low Blood Pressure

BEETS regulate menstruation. Their high potassium and sodium content provides a good solvent for calcium deposits. They are also helpful in treating low vitality, low blood sugar, and anemia and are excellent, blood building liver tonic and alkalizer. Beet leaves are a good source of magnesium, calcium, and iron. The combination of leaf and root provides the essential elements for maintaining a strong, healthy blood stream.

Helpful in a Number
of Common Ailments

CARROTS, exceedingly rich in vitamin A, are excellent for blood cleansing and as an alkalizer. In the raw, they contain nearly all the minerals and vitamins required by the human body. Soothing, healing and nourishing, they are helpful in protecting the eyes and in treating ulcers, anemia, hay fever, colitis, asthma, emphysema, rheumatic conditions, constipation, digestion, and the entire respiratory tract. They are excellent for diabetics; the sugar in carrots is easily digested. Carrot juice added to milk, preferably raw goat's milk or mother's milk for babies, helps build good teeth and bones and tends to prevent rickets. When taken during the last three months of pregnancy, carrots tend to reduce the hazard of infection after childbirth.

A Good Blood
and Skin Purifier

TOMATOES are an outstanding source of vitamins C and A. A good skin and blood purifier, they are helpful for gall stones, acidosis, sinus trouble, dyspepsia, jaundice, and biliousness. They also tend to decrease urinary acidity.

The Best Natural Diuretic

CUCUMBERS are rated very high as a health food by scientists. The ripe seeds contain a mild diuretic, promoting the flow of urine. The high potassium in cucumbers is helpful in high and low blood pressure. Rich in vitamin C, they are helpful in treating neuritis, fevers, obesity, rheumatism, nervousness, pyorrhea, skin eruptions, and acidosis.

Minimizing Insulin
Requirements

CABBAGE is rich in vitamins A, B, and C. These vitamins, plus a high mineral content, are helpful for kidney and bladder disorders, obesity, functional heart trouble, skin eruptions, scurvy, deficiency diseases of the thyroid and adrenal glands, and constipation. A good blood cleanser and detoxifier, it is a valuable aid to teeth, gums, hair, and bones. Cabbage juice, made only from the loose leaf cabbage (the head cabbage is a poor source of vitamins and minerals), is particularly helpful to those suffering from diabetes in that it has been found to cut down insulin requirements. In instances where cabbage juice causes gastric distress, it is better to use it in connection with carrot juice in the proportion of 1 part cabbage to 3 parts carrot.

A Good
Body Building Food

COCONUTS are considered to be an almost complete food. They are rich in protein, and the protein is readily assimilable and rich in many of the natural amino acids. The high vitamin B content helps materially in digestive disorders. Coconuts are soothing and protective in colitis, gastritis, stomach ulcers, sore throat, liver complaints, nervous exhaustion, indigestion, constipation, and the condition of being underweight. It is a good body building food. Coconut and carrot juice in equal amounts make a delicious, protective, and sustaining food beverage.

A Useful Tonic

PARSLEY is an outstanding source of organic iron, excellent source of chlorophyll, and a good source of calcium. It is the highest vegetable source of vitamin A. It is helpful in menstrual and malarial disorders, anemia, halitosis, nephritis, congested liver, rheumatism, high blood pressure, gall stones, all disorders of the urinary tract, and asthma. Parsley juice should not be taken alone. It is best combined with either celery or carrot juice, 7 parts of celery or carrot to 1 part of parsley.

Helpful in Arthritis

ORANGE is a good source of vitamin C. Three and a half ounces of orange juice contain about 900 International Units of vitamin C. Oranges are an excellent source of calcium and phosphorus. A good blood cleanser, oranges are helpful in high blood pressure, diabetes, arthritis, obesity, scurvy, bone and teeth building, and liver disorders, and tend to reduce acidity of urine. Orange juice for babies from 3 weeks to 6 months is best strained and diluted with an equal amount of luke-warm boiled water. It is best given in the morning and afternoon. Quantities recommended each period: 3 weeks, 1 teaspoon; 4 weeks, 1½ teaspoons; 2 months, 1 tablespoon; 3 months, 1½ tablespoons; 4 to 6 months, 2 tablespoons.

Helpful in
Reducing Diets

GRAPEFRUIT is a fine source of vitamin C. In 3½ ounces of grapefruit juice, there are approximately 650 International Units of vitamin C. Grapefruit contains about 7% fruit sugar. It is helpful in reducing diets, acidosis, gall stones, high blood pressure, sluggish liver, malaria, and poor complexion. It prevents colds, acts as a mild diuretic and mild laxative, and renews vitamin C lost during fevers. Do not use it in cases of colitis or inflammation of digestive tract.

Best for
Mucus Elimination

LEMON contains about 6% citric acid and is a high source of vitamin C. Three and a half ounces of lemon juice contain 1000 International Units of vitamin C. Its citric content helps to minimize the dangers of hemorrhage. It is helpful in colds, gout, jaundice, obesity, rheumatism, and liver disorders. Lemon is an excellent blood cleanser. It is not recommended when inflammatory conditions of the digestive tract or colitis are present.

For external use, lemon juice applied to the skin and allowed to dry is helpful in acne and eczema. As an emergency wash and dressing for wounds, it is a natural antiseptic.

Besides clearing the throat of mucus, the juice of one fresh lemon in warm water daily will tend to reduce your weight and maintain it at a normal level at all times. A case-history is in order here: Mrs. L., a dear friend of the family, has been taking lemon juice in water most of her adult life. She plays tennis daily and skis during the winter months with her husband, son, and daughter-in-law.

Another case-history is that of the late Lily Pons, Metropolitan Opera star. A devotee of lemon, she applied it to her face and body, took it internally most of her life—and never gained a pound.

Helpful in
Cases of Insomnia

ONION is a good antiseptic and excellent source of sulphur. A mild diuretic and phlegm expectorant, it is helpful in sinus trouble, catarrh, colds, insomnia, nervousness, pimples and skin eruptions, and stimulating circulation. Onion juice is not taken alone; it is better to use a small amount mixed with celery juice, about 8 parts celery to 1 part onion. Onion is recommended for patients troubled with cystitis or dyspepsia.

Helpful in Bronchitis

PINEAPPLE contains about 12% fruit sugar. The high chlorine content is a digestive aid. It is antiseptic and healing. A gland regulator, it is helpful in dyspepsia, sore throat, bronchitis, obesity, goitre, tumors, catarrh, arthritis, high blood pressure, and diphtheria. It tends to reduce the acidity of urine. It is a mild diuretic and helps in normalizing menstruation.

A Blood Purifier

TURNIP is rich in vitamins A and C. Three and a half ounces of turnip juice contain 1000 International Units of vitamin C. It is a splendid source of organic calcium, and a good source of phosphorus, iron, and sulphur. Turnip leaves are high in chlorophyll. A blood purifier, turnip is helpful in anemia, high blood pressure, sluggish liver, acidosis, poor appetite, bladder disorders, and bone and tooth building.

Indispensable for
Treating Constipation

SPINACH is a protective food, particularly for the glands. A high source of vitamin A, and rich in chlorophyll, it is helpful in high blood pressure, functional heart trouble, anemia, goitre, acidosis, eyes and optic nerve and muscles, nervous exhaustion, obesity, dyspepsia, neuritis, tumors, and constipation. It is indicated in medical circles that raw spinach juice taken in quantities amounting to about one pint daily has often corrected the most aggravated case of constipation in a short period of time.

The Poor Man's Food

BANANA, known as a "poor man's food," is exceedingly nutritious. It contains a high percentage of potassium, a great healer. It keep muscles in tone, and is important for the functioning of liver and kidneys. Contrary to what some people think, the banana will not cause corpulence.

Cell Growth Normalizer

ASPARAGUS, rich in iodine, sulphur, and silicon, contains a good supply of proteins known as "histones," which are believed to be active in controlling cell growth. For that reason, it is believed asparagus can be said to contain a substance known as Cell Growth Normalizer. That accounts for its action on cancer and in acting as a general body tonic.

Asparagus contains a wealth of vitamin A, vitamin C, and the B-Complex vitamins. It also contains such vital minerals as calcium, phosphorus, iron, iodine, sulphur, and silicon and is a good supply of proteins.

A Simple Precaution

If at any time during these nine days you should feel weak or dizzy, and the chances are you won't, take a tablespoon of honey. Also take a calcium concentrate in some form each day to assure a sufficient supply of this important mineral.

Calcium for Good Health

Most people are apt to suffer from a shortage of calcium. A loss of body energy is directly associated with a shortage of calcium. It has long been known that weakness of body and nerves, a below-par condition, and even serious disease are inevitable results of calcium starvation. It has been proven that a shortage of calcium in the diet causes a serious loss of potential body energy. Calcium deficiency decreases the ability of the body to convert food into energy. About 25% of the food's potential energy—and 23% of its protein value—is wasted when calcium is lacking. This makes us realize just how dependent we are on calcium for good health. There is no substitute for it, especially with its associated factors of phosphorus and vitamin D. Calcium concentrates, usually in the form of calcium lactate, are available in health food stores and some supermarkets.

Foods to Omit

During the entire nine days, you should eat no oils, fats, starches, or meats. These foods can prevent or handicap the cleansing effect.

THE
NINE-DA Y INNER CLEANSING AND BLOOD WASH
DA Y BY DA Y

FIRST DAY

Eat only fresh vegetables and fruits, raw and cooked. The more raw food that is eaten, the better.

Take at night, a glassful of Garlic Broth made of the following:

Cut fine six cloves of raw garlic. Cook for seven minutes in a small vessel in one third glass of water. Pour the cooked garlic and broth into an 8 ounce glass and fill the glass with skimmed milk. Goat's milk is best. Drink it before retiring.

Take the minimum daily requirement of calcium lactate in the mid-afternoon.

SECOND DAY

Repeat the entire procedure of the first day.

THIRD DAY

Repeat the entire procedure of the first and second day.

FOURTH DAY

Take an 8 ounce glass of sauerkraut juice first thing on an empty stomach. This in most cases produces a good elimination. It also supplies lactic acid, which aids the growth of friendly flora. If the elimination does not take place, follow up one half hour later with an 8 ounce glass of warm fresh grapefruit juice, or take an *herbal* laxative or an enema.

Continue with fresh fruits and vegetables.

Take the minimum daily requirement of calcium lactate in the mid-afternoon.

FIFTH DAY

Repeat the procedure of the fourth day, with sauerkraut juice, etc.

Continue with fresh fruits and vegetables.

Take the minimum daily requirement of calcium lactate in mid-afternoon.

THE SECRET WEAPON AGAINST DISEASE

Take the "Blood Wash" by starting the day with a quart of fresh orange juice.

Take a quart of grape juice (unsweetened) around noon time. Use fresh grape juice when in season.

Take a quart of pineapple juice (unsweetened), fresh if available, around 3 o'clock in the afternoon.

Finish the day with a quart of fresh orange juice in the evening.

The juices should be taken at intervals until they are consumed, and they should be sipped through a straw.

SIXTH DAY

Repeat the procedure of the fourth and fifth days, with sauerkraut juice, etc.

Take the minimum daily requirement of calcium lactate in mid-afternoon.

Eat an abundance of green salads, the greener the better. The dressing should consist of pure apple cider vinegar, honey, paprika, and some water. Shake well and serve cold.

Drink an abundance of green vegetable juices, the greener the better.

The following green vegetables are recommended: celery, lettuce, spinach, parsley, cucumber, onion, cabbage, rhubarb, and papaya. (Although it is a fruit, papaya is included because of its remarkable therapeutic qualities.)

SEVENTH DAY

Take the minimum daily requirement of calcium lactate in the mid-afternoon.

Eat an abundance of green salads, the greener the better. The dressing is to consist of sesame oil, pure apple cider vinegar, honey, paprika, and some water. Shake well and serve cold.

Drink an abundance of green vegetable juices, the greener the better.

The following green vegetables are recommended: celery, lettuce, spinach parsley, cucumber, onion, cabbage, and rhubarb, as well as papaya.

EIGHTH DAY

Continue with fresh fruits and vegetables.

Take the minimum daily requirement of calcium lactate in mid-afternoon.

Drink all you can of the following fresh juices: orange, grapefruit, apple, papaya, pineapple, coconut, blackberry, and cranberry.

If you are troubled with arthritis, ulcers, acidosis, colitis, emphysema, heartburn, psoriasis, or hay fever, replace the citrus juices with alkaline juices such as apple, papaya, coconut, and acidophilus milk (which is highly alkaline).

NINTH DAY

Continue with fresh fruits and vegetables.

Take the minimum daily requirement of calcium lactate in the mid-afternoon.

Drink all you can of the following fresh vegetable juices: carrot and celery (best combined), parsley and spinach (combined), cabbage, and cucumber, as well as papaya.

Your Path of Rejuvenation

Now you have started on the path of rejuvenation and formed new food habits. There are certain important rules which will help in attaining them. The following should be adhered to:

Eat only young, tender vegetables. If meat is eaten, limit it to once a week, and make sure it is young and lean. Eat broiled beef liver twice a week, fowl twice a week (without the skin), and seafood three time a week. Limit starchy foods severely, especially if you are over 40. Omit white flour and sugar entirely from your diet. Instead, eat an interesting chemical meal which contains all the necessary elements. Large, green salads, with dressing made of sesame oil, fresh apple cider vinegar, honey, paprika, and some water, should be eaten regularly. Don't stuff yourself with bread. One slice with each meal is sufficient. Whole grain, wheat germ, whole wheat, and soya breads are recommended. Eat bran for roughage. Drink 6 to 8 glasses of distilled or spring water daily. Don't drink water during meals. A cup of plain yogurt before retiring is a must. Drink a glassful of fresh lemon juice (one lemon) in warm water three times daily. This has proven to be most effective in the elimination of mucus and keeping your weight normal. For TV and in-between snacks, eat fresh fruit, dates, figs, apricots, raisins, and nuts. Drink two glasses of buttermilk daily.

Foods to Avoid

The foods which you are not to eat are: All white flour products, any and all products made from white sugar, hard water, old vegetables, coarse matured meats, pork, muscle meats, excessively fatty foods, salt, food high in animal fats, adulterated foods, carbonated drinks, processed foods, alcoholic beverages, coffee, tea, rich desserts, ice cream, sweets of all kinds, condiments of all kinds, sauces, gravies, saccharin, synthetic sweeteners, synthetic pills, drugs in the form of laxatives and sedatives, and, especially, homogenized milk, which is highly mucus forming—or any cow's milk, as cows are not immune from tuberculosis, brucellosis, and other ailments. There is no better milk for infants than mother's milk; the next best is raw goat's milk. Skimmed milk and non-fat milk are acceptable.

The growth principle in foods is of great importance. The more *youthful foods* are eaten, the greater the supply of elements from which the body can build *young cells*. The softening properties of distilled water and of vegetable and fruit juices are quickly proved by those who follow the "Nine-Day Inner Cleansing and Blood Wash for Renewed Youthfulness and Health"—the Ever-Young Diet.

Put yourself on a program of regular but simple exercise. Walking and deep breathing are the most acceptable, also bicycling and swimming.

2

Four Natural
Blood-Washing Foods
with
Healing Power

During my years of research and clinical observation, I have singled our four foods that play an important part in healing, curing, and preventing disease.

If I mention blackstrap molasses, cider vinegar, honey, and garlic, you might say, "I know all about them." But you really don't until you read a number of the case histories and recent opinions of medical doctors, nutritionists, scientists, and researchers. Although *one* case history cannot prove a theory no matter how positive the results, molasses has *repeatedly* cured the same kind of disease.

Blackstrap Molasses: Nature's Curative Wonder-Food

If there has ever been a food that was ignored in direct proportion to its prophylactic and curative properties, that food is unsulphured blackstrap molasses. It is truly a wonder-food of nature. No home should ever be without it.

An Unheralded Cancer Fighter

Children should be given a teaspoonful of molasses daily, either straight or with water. Not only will it close the door on cancer in general, but it is especially helpful in cases of leukemia (cancer of the blood), which afflicts some children.

Avoiding Breast Cancer

Adults, particularly women, who have breast cancer or may be prone to it, should take a tablespoon of unsulphured blackstrap molasses twice daily, plus vitamins E, C, and A. (Men are also prone to breast cancer, although it is not as common.)

To prevent and heal breast cancer (among other things), it is also of paramount importance to employ the "Nine-Day Inner Cleansing and Blood Wash" twice yearly, six months apart. This cleanses and purifies the body of stored-up poisonous wastes (toxins) that have accumulated and formed a lining around the intestinal wall over the years, leading to disease. The basic principle of the nine-day program, "healing the body first," applies to breast cancer as well as other diseases.

The Difficulty in
Isolating Cancer Cells

A stagnant cellular condition, especially with billions of live cells in the body, makes it extremely difficult to isolate the impaired cells, and contributes, in large measure, to cancerous conditions, including breast cancer. Molasses can play an important role in preventing a stagnant cellular condition. Cyril Scott, a noted English medical writer and one of the most leading authorities on blackstrap molasses, maintains that an important constituent of molasses is phosphoric acid; a combined deficiency of this and potassium in the human body "causes a general breakdown of the cells, especially those of the brain and nerves."

The widespread use of wonder drugs, patent foods, and patent medicines does more harm than good in many cases. There is nothing whatever patent about molasses. The naturopaths and the less orthodox physicians are fully aware of its curative and prophylactic properties. Think it over seriously, and then get to work at once. I can't help being disturbed when I think of breast cancer increasingly taking its toll of lives all over the world.

The Value of Molasses in Connection with Cancer

It is belived that the late Dr. Forbes Ross was the first English doctor to draw attention to the prophylactic and curative properties in molasses. He pointed out that workers on sugar cane plantations, who were constantly sucking the crude sugar in sugar cane, seldom if ever were known to suffer from cancer. He attributed this to the large percentage of potassium salts in unrefined sugar cane, his argument being that the cause of cancer was a deficiency of potash in the human cells and blood. Dr. Ross's numerous cures of cancer, together with the book he wrote on the subject, did not, at the time, receive the recognition they deserved. However, several eminent physicians of various schools have since come to uphold his views.

Highly Rich in Iron and Calcium

Blackstrap molasses, gram for gram, contains more iron than any other food except for pig's liver and brewer's yeast. It contains five times more calcium than milk. It is an abundant source of all the B vitamins and contains relatively large amounts of copper, potassium and phosphorus in addition to a sizeable amount of the trace mineral chromium, which has recently been found to be valuable in maintaining proper blood sugar levels. Ten percent of the total content of blackstrap molasses is minerals.

A Case History
Worthy of Note

Cyril Scott's attention was more fully drawn to the curative and prophylactic elements in blackstrap molasses by one of his numerous correspondents, a Mr. James Persson, of Palmerston N., New Zealand. The circumstances are as follows: Some years earlier Mr. Persson was in a state of broken health and unable to do even the lightest work. He was suffering from a growth in the bowels, blocked bronchial tubes, constipation, indigestion, pyorrhea, sinus trouble, and weak nerves. In addition to this array of symptoms, he was losing weight, and his hair had turned white. Despite consultation of doctors and specialists, his condition was steadily getting worse. Then one day he heard of a Mr. S. who happened to be a neighbor of the postman. Mr. Persson got these details from the postman: Mr. S. had suffered from an inoperable growth of the bowels; he had been opened up by the surgeon and then simply stitched up again because his condition was regarded as so hopeless that even the idea of surgical interference was abandoned. He was discharged from the hospital and given only seven weeks to live. However, an aquaintance convinced him to try the effect of taking molasses. Astonishingly, instead of dying within seven weeks he finally made a complete recovery. On hearing of this remarkable cure, Mr. Persson decided to try the treatment on himself. And not only did the growth in his bowels disappear, together with all the other troubles (and this after seven years of suffering), but his hair, which was white when he started the treatment, actually regained its original color and assumed a more healthy appearance. It should be mentioned that Mr. Persson was over sixty at the time.

A Great Demand for Molasses

Having proved for himself the curative value of molasses, he resolved to supply the aliment to those suffering from various ailments, including growths. When Mr. S's cure and Mr. Persson's own cure became known, the demand for molasses was such that Mr. Persson was at one time supplying a ton a month.

Growths are serious conditions for which the orthodox medico can only suggest radium or the knife. But, among the numerous cases cured solely by molasses-therapy are: growths of the uterus, growths of the breast, intestinal growths, and malignant growths of the tongue.

Other Case Histories

One man, whom we will call Mr. X, had a fibroid growth of the tongue and was in such an advanced condition that he was unable to speak. As treatment, he repeatedly held molasses in his mouth and also took it internally; the growth went away and the man was cured.

According to Mr. Persson and to reports received by him, tumors in various parts of the body have withered away without any other measures than taking molasses internally and using it in the form of poultices.

Incidentally, I should mention a fibroid case of my own. Several years ago a wart the size of a pea developed on my left wrist. I knew that a skin disease is an attempt on the part of nature to rid the body of certain poisons; and to suppress that attempt by smearing on ointments is a sure way to drive these poisons back into the body. So I applied poultices of blackstrap molasses to the unsightly wart, renewing them daily, and took molasses internally at the same time so as to get rid of the condition of the blood and tissues that was primarily responsible for the disorder. The wart gradually diminished, and to my great surprise it dropped off completely in about two weeks without leaving a blemish.

Strangely enough, a wart also made an unwelcomed appearance on the right shoulder of my wife. This one was the size of a flattened pea. The same molasses-therapy was used. In this case it took about four weeks for the wart to disappear, largely because of its size.

A Doctor Recovers from Ulcers

In cases of ulcers and ulcerations, Mr. Persson reports that they have been cured by molasses. He cites the case of a certain doctor in New Zealand who was so much afflicted with ulcers that his own skill proved insufficient to cure them. In fact, the doctor was very ill and would doubtless have remained so had he not heard of the molasses-treatment and been open-minded enough to try it. The result was that, after taking molasses for a period of time, all his ulcers vanished and he was restored to excellent health.

According to Cyril Scott, practitioners of the Biochemic System of Medicine concur that ulcers do not develop unless there is a deficiency of certain mineral salts in the blood and tissues. As molasses, if taken over the requisite time, makes good that deficiency, it is not surprising to hear that gastric ulcers have also yielded to the treatment.

Coughing Up Rotten Growths

Mr. Persson further reports that many sufferers, after taking molasses for some time, coughed up rotten growths. Among others, he gives the case of a man said to be suffering from cancer of the gullet. This unfortunate man had to be fed by the means of a tube. After treating himself with molasses, he coughed up a rotten lump about the size of a small egg.

Recovering from a Breast Growth

A Mrs. M, suffering from a breast growth, was given two months to live. After employment of molasses-therapy, the growth disappeared, and she was perfectly well. Many months elapsed. No recurrence.

A "Miracle" Recovery from Two Strokes

The general supposition is that when a person has had two strokes the third one will be fatal. And yet it need not be so—or at any rate not always—as the following case history reveals: Mr. K, an elderly man, had had two strokes and was completely paralyzed on one side of his body. He then tried molasses-therapy. The result was that he recovered the use of all his limbs and became completely fit, much to the astonishment of his doctor. This case has been selected out of many others because it happens to have been a particularly bad one.

Cases of Sinus Trouble Yield
to Molasses-Therapy

It is not surprising to learn from Cyril Scott that cases of sinus trouble have yielded to molasses-therapy. For this complaint, the substance must be taken internally and a mild solution of it used as a nasal douche; the same measures have also been very beneficial in cases of nasal catarrh and antrum trouble.

Beneficial in Menopause

Molassses-therapy has proved of enormous value to women during menopause. Menopause is said to be—and often is—a very difficult time for women. But in a large number of cases, this can be attributed to years of eating wrong foods and a deficiency of mineral salts and vitamins.

Healthy and Easy Pregnancy

Many prospective mothers who have taken molasses during the term of pregnancy have not only had easy confinements but have given birth to healthy infants.

Overcoming Anemia

Cases of anemia, in many instances "pernicious" anemia, have been cured by taking molasses. The orthodox treatment of anemia—which consists largely in the administration of an iron preparation in large doses for a long time—is not only unsatisfactory but is often accompanied by digestive disturbances. The reason is obvious to all naturopaths: iron and calcium should be absorbed from a natural food and not from a medicinal preparation, however scientific it is supposed to be.

Beneficial in
Varicose Veins

Some naturopaths have been using molasses for varicose veins. The treatment is perfectly rational. When taken internally it makes good that deficiency of mineral salts which is the prime cause of this annoying and often debilitating condition.

Overcoming Erysipelas

A case of erysipelas was cured with molasses; and the doctor in attendance advised the patient to continue taking the aliment in view of its beneficial result.

Speedy Recovery from
Cancer of the Knee

A man with a large lump below the knee, diagnosed as cancer, decided to have it extirpated. But prior to the operation he was induced to take the molasses treatment. The subsequent and speedy healing of the wound was commented on by his physicians.

A Case History of My Own

When surgery has been resorted to for one reason or another, the healing processes have been greatly facilitated and accelerated when the paient has taken molasses treatment prior to and following the operation. Strange as it may seem, here is an obvious and instructive case of my own.

Several years ago I was operated on for the removal of my prostate gland at Roosevelt Hospital in New York City. After several tests and x-rays, the physicians in attendance were astonished to learn that I was otherwise in perfect health. The regular employment of the ever-reliable "Nine-Day Inner Cleansing and Blood Wash" was largely responsible for the remarkable condition I was in particularly at my age. The medicos looked askance and raised their eyes when they were made aware of this.

Much to the surprise of the surgeon who operated on me, I was in the recovery room for just a short while after the operation, while other patients remained there overnight. I was discharged from the hospital in perfect condition after a short recuperative period.

Before the operation, I went through agony for about a year, trying to avoid surgery by using the following program of therapy: massages of the prostate gland three times a week by a chiropractor, hot sitz baths daily, hot packs daily (applying hot towels to the crotch and lower abdomen), and chewing parsley daily. Nothing helped. I got some temporary relief in being able to urinate, but that's about all. And all during that time I was being tortured with catheterization each time I had a spell of prostatitis (not being able to urinate). No one has even been able to find the cause of prostatitis. We do know that men past 45 are prone to it no matter how healthy they may be. Seven out of every ten men in that age group become afflicted with it.

Don't Make the
Same Mistake I Made

My advice is that once you have become a victim of prostatitis have the prostate gland removed at once—surgically.

We have yet to find any other cure for it.

The Most Convenient Way
of Taking Molasses

The most convenient way of taking molasses is before meals. The dosage is one teaspoonful, which should be melted in half a cup of hot water. Then add cold water to make about two-thirds of a cup. Drink this warm. For children, give half the dosage. The molasses can be taken straight, but hot water should be drunk immediately afterwards. Some people, however, find the latter method unsuited to them. The patient must use his own judgement and adapt the method to his individual idiosyncracies. Persons with delicate stomachs, who find a teaspoonful too much at one time, should take smaller doses several times during the day. The water should, of course, never be too hot—never hotter than a temperature in which one can comfortably bear to put one's finger. It is the utmost folly to drink any beverage scaldingly hot, like some persons drink tea. Another point is that the molasses-and-water mixture should not be gulped down like nasty medicine so as to produce flatulence, but should be sipped and tasted like connoisseurs taste good wines.

Cider Vinegar: A Wonder Beverage

Cyril Scott, in a treatise on cider vinegar, draws attention to the highly valuable properties contained in cider vinegar, and the number of ailments that will automatically disappear after taking that beverage in the prescribed manner. It can justly be called a wonder-beverage.

The Safest Cure
for Obesity

If cider vinegar is taken from one to three times a day, during meals or not, reduction of weight without dieting will be achieved permanently. The cider vinegar will burn up the surplus fat. It is nature's great health promoter and safest cure for obesity, which by the way is not looked upon as a disease in the ordinary sense of the word.

Why a Common Table Fluid Is So Beneficial

It may be asked why this common table fluid should be so beneficial. And the very simple and self-evident answer is that it is made of apples, which are perhaps the most health-giving fruits that exist. "An apple a day keeps the doctor away" is no empty slogan, for apples contain some very important chemical ingredients. A second question might be, what are the functions of cider vinegar—exactly what does it do? Stated in brief: it favors oxidation of the blood; it tends to prevent intestinal putrefaction; it regulates calcium metabolism; it retards the onset of old age; it renders the urine normal, thus counteracting a too frequent urge to urinate; it affects the blood, making it of the right consistency; it regulates menstruation (and hence is very beneficial to women); and it promotes digestion because cider vinegar bears a closer resemblance to the digestive juices than does any other liquid.

Modifying the Desire to Over-Eat

In severe cases, cider vinegar can be taken with the chief meals of the day, as well as in the morning. The beverage should be sipped so that the entire glass is emptied by the time the meal is finished. This, in addition to its other effects, modifies the desire to over-eat and promotes digestion.

The method of treatment is as follows: Take two teaspoons of cider vinegar in a glass of water on rising in the morning. To be effective, this practice must be continued over a long period. Obesity cannot be expected to vanish within 24 hours; nor is desirable that it should, as the skin requires ample time to re-adjust itself.

Dr. D. C. Jarvis, M.D. of Vermont, has furnished Cyril Scott with the following case histories, though many more could be selected from his own casebook, and from the archives of Vermont Rural Medicine.

How She Lost Her "Stenographer's Seat"

Patient, 31 years old. When she started the cider vinegar treatment, she weighted 148 pounds. Most of her bulk was in the posterior, and she developed what is called "stenographer's seat." By taking the diluted cider vinegar every morning before breakfast (not at any other times), she gradually lost her excess weight, and her "stenographer's seat" completely disappeared. Nevertheless, she continues to take the beverage every morning, with the gratifying result that she can eat what she likes, and the amount that her appetite demands, without putting on weight.

How She Improved Her Heart Condition

Patient, age 50. She had to give up work because of a bad heart. In 1945 she weighed 208 pounds. She then started to take cider vinegar with her meals, and two years later she had reduced her weight to 164 pounds, although she had made no alteration in her diet. As she lost weight her heart condition materially improved.

What should be stressed is that *ordinary vinegar* must *not* be used, as it does not contain the properties of vinegar made from apples and in the long run would certainly prove harmful.

How to Reduce Hemophilia
to a Minimum

Hemophilia is a condition which has baffled most therapeuticians, and persons suffering from this disorder are called "bleeders." The general verdict is that nothing can be done for them; consequently they live in dread of the most trifling accident, such as the cutting of a finger or a mishap while shaving. It is an impressive fact that the taking of cider vinegar in the manner already indicated favors that clotting of the blood which fails to occur in the case of "bleeders." The reason is to be found in the improved metabolism which the vinegar brings about.

Excessive bleeding can be reduced to a minimum in the case of an operation, and the healing process greatly quickened, if the patient takes a teaspoonful or more of cider vinegar in a half or whole glass of water with each meal two or more weeks before the operation and continues to take it for two or more weeks after the operation.

How to Put a Stop to
Frequent Nose-Bleeding

In cases of frequent nose-bleeding due to some indeterminate cause, a drink of the vinegar beverage with each meal will soon put a stop to the trouble.

How to Cure a
Sore Throat Rapidly

Sore throats, even of the streptococcus type, can be cured with astonishing rapidity—often in one day—by taking cider vinegar as a gargle. The treatment consists of adding one teaspoonful of the vinegar to a glass of water. Every hour the sufferer should gargle with one mouthful of the mixture. A second mouthful should be taken, gargled with, and then swallowed. This procedure should be repeated every 60 minutes during waking hours, or even at night if the patient cannot sleep. As soon as the soreness has improved, the intervals of gargling, etc., can be lengthened to two hours. When the patient is cured, it is advisable to use the gargle after each meal for a few days to insure that the trouble will not return.

How You Can Recover from a Tickling Cough

Towards the end of a cold, many people suffer from that annoying and sleep-preventing irritation we call a "tickling cough." In many cases neither lozenges nor other measures have any result. Most cough-mixtures that doctors prescribe contain a drug to deaden the nerve, and drugs in the long run are harmful; on the other hand, the cider vinegar treatment is both harmless and effective. All that is necessary is to place at the bedside a glass of water to which one or two teaspoonfuls of the vinegar have been added. As the tickling sensation is felt, take a few swallows of the mixture. The "tickle" will rapidly disappear, leaving the sufferer able to sleep again.

How You Can Recover from Laryngitis in 7 Hours

For the distressing condition of acute laryngitis, the effect of the cider vinegar treatment is almost miraculous. The dosage is one teaspoonful of the vinegar to half a glass of water, to be taken every hour for seven hours. In most cases, the sufferer will be talking normally after the seventh dose.

Helpful in a
Mild Type of Asthma

In cases of that mild type of asthma which only occurs during the night, and where the wheezing interferes with sleep, take one tablespoon of cider vinegar in a glass of water; this should be taken in sips for half an hour. The patient should wait another half hour and then repeat the procedure. If the wheezing should still persist, though it usually is gone by then, a second glass of the same mixture should be sipped. Deep breathing should be practiced gradually. If practiced daily, in combination with the cider vinegar treatment, it will most likely effect a cure.

How You May Restore Your
Mental and Physical Vigor

It has been found that the diluted vinegar beverage will restore vigor, both mental and physical, in cases where it has already been lost. And when I speak of mental vigor, I include a marked improvement of the memory. Observers have been quite astonished to see how forgetfulness in old people partially or wholly disappears through the practice of taking one teaspoonful of cider vinegar in a whole glass of water, either with meals or between meals, whichever method is preferred or suits the individual best.

How You May Overcome Heartburn
and Digestive Troubles

If the cider vinegar is taken with meals in the prescribed manner, it will seldom cause indigestion; as I have already pointed out, it bears a closer resemblance to the gastric juices than does any other fluid. It is no surprise that vinegar made from apples is very helpful towards the cure of many digestive troubles if taken as already indicated.

Unless due to some serious disorder of the stomach, or to the habit of swallowing air, eructations (belching) can be cured or greatly lessened by taking the cider vinegar beverage with the chief meals of the day. As for heartburn, that burning sensation which may occur after meals—sometimes one or two hours after—this often disappears entirely after resorting to the beverage (or at any rate it is greatly reduced).

How to Relieve Yourself of Frequent Urination

If urine is either too acid or too alkaline, the troublesome and embarrassing necessity for frequent urination occurs in both sexes. In the case of younger people, it is often a matter of the urine being too alkaline, whereas in older people the cause is usually found in the fact that the urine is too acid. But whether too acid or too alkaline, it can, according to Vermont Folk Medicine, be brought back to normal if the cider vinegar beverage (two teaspoonfuls of vinegar to the glass of water) is taken with the chief meals of the day— except in cases of serious disorders of the urinary tract, which need special treatment. Elderly men will often find this treatment very helpful in relieving the frequent desire to pass urine during the night.

Cider vinegar has also been found to be beneficial to women after childbirth and to women during or after menstruation.

Honey: A Food for Healing

Honey has been considered to be a perfect food since ancient times. Not more than one hundreth part of it is wastage. Day by day we are learning more about the elements in honey that are essential to physical well-being. Truly, it is a food for the gods! No household should ever be without it. It is a most effective remedy for insomnia, emphysema, shortness of breath, sinusitis, asthma, and chronic fatigue. Combined with the cider vinegar treatment, it is most beneficial to those suffering from various heart troubles, hay fever, colitis, arthritis, neuritis, and many of other common ailments. The cider vinegar and honey combination is often helpful in promoting sound, healthy sleep.

Rich in Vitamins and Minerals

Honey contains practically all of the vitamins. However, the minerals in honey are even more important. It contains potassium (prevents growths), copper (good for the liver), sulphur (the blood purifier), iron (very important), magnesium, calcium, sodium, silica, and chlorine.

How to Rid Your Body of Deadly Germs

Years of research have uncovered the fact that honey posesses natural laxative properties and is one of nature's most powerful germ killers. Two teaspoons of honey, at the least, should form part of the daily diet of ailing persons who wish to get well—and of all well persons who desire to maintain their health.

Overcoming Gastric Ulcers

Honey is not sufficiently appreciated in this country—except by naturopaths and the like—despite the fact that Russian medico-scientists have shown that it will cure a condition as serious as gastric ulcers.

The Valuable
Elements in Honey

In order to awaken some enthusiasm for honey in the general reader, I will mention the valuable elements it contains. To begin with, it contains vitamin B-1, called thiamine, which is to be found in the husks of cereal grains and is therefore lacking in white bread. Secondly, it contains vitamin B-2, called riboflavin, which is to be found in yeast, milk, and meat, and also in fish and liver. Thirdly, it contains vitamin C (ascorbic acid), to be found in fresh fruits (oranges, etc.) and in fresh greenstuffs. To complete the list, honey also contains pantothenic acid, pyridoxine and nicotinic acid, the latter being part of the B-2 complex. When there is a complete lack of B-1 in the diet, that grave disease called beri-beri ensues. Where there is a shortage but not a complete lack of the thiamine, muscular weakness and heart weakness are frequently the result. As for vitamin C, a complete lack of it results in scurvy, and a partial lack of it in swellings and inflammation of the gums, loss of teeth, hemorrhages under the skin, and other serious conditions.

Dr. G. N. W. Thomas of Edinburgh, in an article about honey in the British medical journal *Lancet*, writes:

> In heart weakness I have found honey to have a marked effect in reviving the heart action and keeping the patients alive. I suggest that honey should be given for general physical repair and, above all, for heart failure.

The treatment, especially for heart trouble, is as follows: Two teaspoons of honey in a glass of water at each meal, whether added to the beverage or taken separately.

Garlic: The Three-Thousand-Year-Old Miracle Medicine

Garlic was known and used over three thousand years ago and has been publicized, recorded and mentioned in medical books since the advent of printing. It is the oldest known "home remedy." It has long been used to rid the body of parasites and in the healing of disease. According to an old news item, "in test tube experiments Virile bacilli that can be killed only after hours of boiling in water die, after one hour of exposure to garlic fumes."

Garlic, too, is a wonder-food. And, like molasses and cider vinegar, it has been largely ignored.

Avail Yourself of the Remarkable Restorative Powers of Garlic

Garlic's almost miraculous antiseptic power is an aid in high blood pressure, asthma, emphysema, colds, gas, gall stones, bronchitis, infections, hardening of the arteries, mucus, elimination, sinus trouble, and many other maladies. It has been widely used in restoring masculine vigor and putting pow wow in your sex life. It is as effective as tolbutamide (an oral drug for diabetics) in clearing the blood stream of excess glucose. It has remarkable preventive powers and healing powers and offers protection against heart disease.

A California study has found that garlic extract will kill five separate species of mosquitoes, and one study with mice brought the discovery that the antibiotic component of garlic oil can inhibit the growth of tumor cells. It is a good plant source of trace elements, iron, potassium, sulphur, iodine, zinc, manganese, phosphorus, copper, fluorine, and vitamins B, C, and D. While it is best in its natural form, raw, it can be obtained at health food stores in capsule form.

Spain's Mortality Rate Is Low
Compared to the U.S.

People in Spain are big garlic eaters. The death rate in Spain from heart disease is less than one-third that in the United States. Italians also eat a lot of garlic, and they, too, have a comparatively low cardiac mortality rate.

How Mr. C Recovered from
Dangerously High Blood Pressure

Mr. C suffered from dangerously high blood pressure of 312. In 1964 he had a heart attack. After taking two capsules of garlic before each meal for about a year and a half, his blood pressure was reduced to an amazing low of 147. He had heart failure in 1975, and his pressure remained at 147.

How Miss M Recovered
from Mild Diabetes

Miss M, diagnosed as having mild diabetes, was told by her doctor she would have to take an oral drug if her blood sugar didn't drop. After taking a 5 grain garlic capsule along with her vitamins and brewer's yeast after each nutritional meal, her blood sugar fell to normal and no drug was needed or prescribed.

How a Patient Recovered from
Diarrhea and High Blood Pressure

A patient had suffered from diarrhea ever since the surgeon had removed hemorrhoids for him. After taking 3 garlic perles a day for a few months, his diarrhea and high blood pressure disappeared.

How Mrs. R's Little Daughter Recovered from Sinus Problems

When Mrs. R's young daughter was suffering from sinus trouble, Mrs. R gave her 2 garlic tablets about every four hours. The next morning, after having taken about six tablets the previous day, the child woke up with a clear head and felt fine.

The diligent use of molasses, with its extensive curative properties, cider vinegar, with its prophylactic properties, honey, with its healing powers, and garlic, with its remarkable preventive and healing powers, will aid tremendously in "healing the body" by way of the "Nine-Day Inner Cleansing and Blood Wash for Renewed Youthfulness and Health."

3

The "Miraculous"
Healing Power
of
Internal Baths

Internal baths are a mighty and powerful weapon for healing and warding off disease. You can cure almost any disease you have permanently and by yourself, right in your own home, the "natural" way.

No dangerous drugs or injections with their serious side effects. No costly medical treatments or tedious regimens. No pains. This system can be life-saving when illness strikes. It will nip some diseases in the bud, reduce ailments by aiding in the healing processes, overcome constipation and diarrhea in no time at all, slim you down without dieting or the use of drugs, overcome shortness of breath, aid in the healing processes of heart trouble, and keep you alive when you have a heart attack or stroke.

Internal baths (bowel flushing enemas) will cleanse the body of stored up poisonous wastes (toxins) and foreign matter that have accumulated and formed a lining around the intestinal wall since childhood. Retention of poisons, caused by sluggish circulation and elimination, will lead to decline in vigor and function, and sooner or later it will lead to the contraction of disease if the poisons are allowed to stagnate.

Dissipating the Possibility of Cancer of the Rectum

In conformity with medical literature in general, I was led to believe that after a bowel movement the lining around the inner rectum wall remains coated with toxic residue that, if allowed to stagnate, may lead to cancer of the rectum—a disease which is increasing at an astonishing rate. With this in mind, I came to the conclusion that bowel flushing enemas are helpful in keeping the inner rectum wall clean of toxic residue.

Wiping your rectum with toilet tissue after a regular bowel movement will not solve the problem. Flushing out the "tiger in your tank" immediately after a bowel movement with two quarts of warm water and a tablespoonful of blackstrap molasses will aid in detoxification and in the healing processes of those suffering from illness.

Bowel flushing enemas are fabulous! They are the most powerful weapons against obesity and produce "impossible" cures at times. They represent a positive way to avoid ever having a heart attack.

Elimination of Digested Food Before Putrefaction Sets In

There may be those who claim that enemas will weaken the patient. I have been taking bowel flushing enemas every day for the past 30 years, and have never had any weakening effects whatsoever.

What is most important is the fact an enema provides further cleansing of digested food that at times remains in the upper intestine as a result of an *incomplete* bowel movement. If allowed to stagnate, this will cause putrefaction. I doubt if there is a person who would be aware of this, unless he had experienced, by trial and error—as I did—such a vital discovery. People generally feel that once they have had a regular bowel movement they have done their duty; few are aware of the serious consequences that will possibly arise from *incomplete* bowel movements.

Give yourself time to have a complete—and I mean complete—bowel movement each morning. Rushing through your morning chores and telling yourself you don't have the time to go to the toilet may be paving the way to serious consequences. Allowing toxic food from the day before to remain in the stomach, and adding breakfast and maybe lunch to it, will put an extra demand on the heart. Acute indigestion has put many a businessman in the obituary columns long before his time.

I am reminded of an attorney I was personally acquainted with who had never had a heart condition, yet died of a heart attack at the age of 39 because he neglected his health. Had he known better, he could have looked after his health first—and that extra buck he was after would have come later, while he was still alive.

Bowel Flushing Enemas
Pay Off in Dividends

Mae West, super star of stage and screen in the 40's, was proof-positive of the "miraculous" effects of bowel flushing enemas. She lived a full life well into her late eighties. She gave herself an enema every day, sometimes two a day. She believed that our insides should be as clean as our outsides, and said "that's what prevents old age." She added that when the insides deteriorate, that's when old age sets in; when you're clean inside you have energy. Look at me, she said, I never stop. And my age isn't a secret. She was in the habit of taking enemas daily all of her adult life.

She drank only bottled spring water, and she wouldn't touch anything canned or frozen because frozen food is dead food, and, according to Mae West, the preservatives in the cans may be good for the cans, but they're not good for you.

Once a month, she fasted for three days running. She did not use salt in her food, maintaining that there's enough salt in everything. She did not smoke or drink. She did not eat lunch—she just ate fresh fruit every hour or two. She nibbled on about five or six unsalted almonds a day. Edgar Cayce told her they're a good preventive for cancer. She went for years without having a cold. She was quite a lady. If you will follow her mode of living, you'll live to be one-hundred-and-five, and maybe more.

A Case History
Worthy of Note

Will Durant, famous American professor of philosophy and prominent author, kept up a punishing lecture schedule until 1957, when hypertension forced him to quit. On one of his trips, he met Dr. John Harvey Kellog, the Battle Creek, Michigan nutritionist, and Durant became converted to vegetarianism and daily enemas. Dr. Kellog developed the first Kellog cereals, and was connected with the company at that time.

Durant swore by the Kellog regimen and said it cured him of arthritis and kept him healthy well into his nineties.

Some doctors will tell you not to worry if you go 3 days without a bowel movement. Some will even go so far as to say not to worry whenever you go a week or two without a bowel movement. Little do such doctors realize that such long periods of accumulation of undigested and uneliminated toxic waste matter make the body prone to a heart attack or stroke.

A Way to Overcome Habitual Use of Harmful Drug Laxatives

People are foolishly resorting to harmful drug laxatives in place of enemas.

Here is a case history that hits home:

My late mother-in-law, Mace MacKibben, was seriously afflicted with persistent constipation and indigestion most of her adult life. I begged her, time and again, to try using bowel flushing enemas, assuring her that such therapy would solve her problems. However, she was unduly stubborn and continued with her laxatives.

Of this you can be sure: there is no such thing as a harmless laxative on the market. The advertised gentle ones are no less destructive than the strong ones. By consistent use, any of them will create a dependency, and in time you are "hooked" and cannot get along without them. A negative reaction brought on by habitual use of laxatives is the gradual desensitization of the colon and anal sphincter; and they are robbed of their natural function.

Due to my mother-in-law taking a well known saline laxative (name withheld) for years, a problem developed which required surgery. The doctor treating her found her case beyond his realm and sent her to a specialist. The specialist found that her colon had become paralyzed. He diagnosed the cause as being the habitual use of this highly recommended laxative. The laxative created a buildup of saline deposits that resulted in a numbing of the organs necessary to propel defecation (commonly termed moving the bowels). The surgery involved the removal of about an inch and a half of the colon. She was never the same after that painful operation. Eventually, she became paralyzed from her hips down.

Outmoding Purgative Medicine

When my generation was young, it was the practice when anything went wrong—a cold, fever, lethargy, ennui, anything that made a change in one's facial expression—to respond with the diagnosis of "the child needs a purge." Until this was outmoded, there were many cases of damaged intestines and unnecessary discomfort. But you cannot censure a person for being ignorant; only for remaining ignorant.

I Hold the Key
to a Locked Bowel

For a natural, fast, effective, and harmless laxative, I recommend an 8 oz. glass of warm sauerkraut juice followed by an 8 oz. glass of warm grapefruit juice. It will clean you out almost instantly.

If your insides have become stagnant with an accumulation of stored-up poisonous waste and foreign matter and the attempt of elimination is unsuccessful, repeat the same process a half hour later.

No enema is required.

I have tried the same laxative remedy on members of my family and friends and relatives who were troubled with constipation and indigestion. It has never failed to work like "magic." It relieved a "locked bowel" of a friend of the family almost immediately.

How to Overcome Obesity
and Live Longer

Gastro-intestinal upsets will vanish completely after you get into the habit of taking bowel flushing enemas daily, as prescribed. You will be able to function physically in a calm and easy manner. The general feeling of "battle fatigue" that obese people usually experience will disappear. You will have a zest for living. You will be able to double your work output.

Persistent obesity will, directly or indirectly, cause shortness of breath and lack of vigor, bring about diseases of all kinds, and shorten your life.

The obvious causes of obesity are over-consumption of fatty, starchy and sugary foods, overeating, snacks between meals, over indulgence in alcoholic beverages, particularly beer, and lack of exercise.

Why Overweight People
Are Prone to Heart Disease

The strain that excess weight places upon the heart has lead the American Heart Association to conduct a vigorous campaign against obesity. It has been noted by the U.S. Public Health Service that heart disease occurs two or three times more frequently in people who are seriously overweight.

Obesity, however, is a far more dangerous problem than even those statistics indicate. Overweight persons not only reduce their day-to-day effectiveness but also increase surgical risks and complicate almost any disease they contract, such as arthritis, diabetes, and hypertension.

Do not, under any circumstance, use diet pills to reduce. So many of them are known to be dangerous to health.

Diet Pills Have "Extremely Limited"
Value in Weight Loss Programs

In December of 1972, the Food and Drug Administration concluded that amphetamine diet pills have "extremely limited" value in weight loss programs, and, because of the volume of these pills disappearing into the illegal drug market—where amphetamines are known as "speed"—the FDA succeeded in forcing drug companies to cut their amphetamine production by 80%.

What to Do for "Quick Weight Loss"

For "quick weight loss," cut out all carbohydrates and fats, and limit yourself to seafood, lean meats, eggs, poultry, cottage cheese, and fresh fruits and vegetables. Drink from six to eight glasses of distilled water a day. Take time to enjoy each meal and chew properly. Gradually accustom your stomach to being satisfied with a little less filling at each sitting. And last, but not least, put yourself on a program of regular but simple exercise. Walking is the most acceptable and can be stimulating to the mind as well as the body.

Begin with a stroll; then, as you feel inclined, increase the cadence of your steps to a comfortable gait. Start to jog after you have taken off some weight—slowly at first. Then work your way carefully up to more strenuous exercises.

You will experience new found joy when you are able to walk up stairs without stopping every few steps to catch your breath, when you can bend over and tie your own shoelace, and especially when you move about with ease.

Method

Hold the enema bag no more than 10 to 12 inches above your head. Fill the bag with one and a half quarts of water—about as hot as your fingers can stand—and allow it to run in slowly. In order that you do not irritate the rectum, use a small tip lubricated with vaseline. You will learn after a while to regulate the flow by contracting or relaxing the intestinal muscles. At times, when I feel that my bowel movement has been complete, I stop the flow of water midway and flush out the lower intestine only. At other times, when I feel my bowel movement has not been complete, I allow the water to flow gently into the upper intestine, retain it for a minute or so, then expel it slowly. This will dislodge the excrement that may have accumulated there, and which, if allowed to remain and stagnate, will cause putrefaction to set it, polluting the blood stream.

The natural and harmless bowel flushing therapy is a "break-through" of utmost importance. It is my own secret discovery, after extensive research and trial by error. Now for the first time, I am making it available to people suffering from illnesses.

Fasting goes hand in hand with bowel flushing enemas. It gives your insides, working all the time, a much needed rest. The longer you go without food, the more waste matter is thrown into the blood stream, which carries it to the various organs of elimination. If this waste matter remains in the blood, we become sick.

A Pleasurable Way of Fasting

Water fasting is a miserable process. Here is a pleasurable method by which you can have all of the results, less the misery of the old way:

Upon rising each morning, take the juice of one fresh lemon in a glass of hot or cold water without sweetening. One hour later, take a glass of fresh orange and fresh grapefruit juice. Repeat this every four hours until bedtime. I have been fasting this way for a great number of years and recommend it highly.

While on the fast, I rest in bed as much as I can and do not over-exert myself or undergo undue strain.

Fasting is not recommended for those suffering from

arthritis, diabetes, cancer, heart trouble, hay fever, emphysema, colitis, and ulcers.

Could You Ask for Anything More?

The "magic" healing power of internal baths is next in importance to the Nine-Day Inner Cleansing and Blood Wash for Renewed Youthfulness and Health.

It will aid the healing processes of disease, ward off cancer, and, at times, produce "impossible" cures if you employ both of the fabulous therapies as prescribed, fasting 2 days every other month, daily using 800 I.U. of Vitamin E, all of the Vitamin C the body can take, 10,000 I.U. of Vitamin A, the major minerals, 3 tablespoons of blackstrap molasses, the juice of one lemon in warm water 3 times daily, and changing your eating habits to nutritional foods. You will never have a sick day in your life! Could you ask for anything more?

DESIRABLE WEIGHTS

WOMEN

Height (with shoes on) 2-inch heels	Small Frame	Medium Frame	Large Frame
4' 10"	92-98	96-107	104-119
11"	94-101	98-110	106-122
5' 0"	96-104	101-113	109-125
1"	99-107	104-116	112-128
2"	102-110	107-119	115-131
3"	105-113	110-122	118-134
4"	108-116	113-126	121-138
5"	111-119	116-130	125-142
6"	114-123	120-135	129-146
7"	118-127	124-139	133-150
8"	122-131	128-143	137-154
9"	126-135	132-147	141-158
10"	130-140	136-151	145-163
11"	134-144	140-155	149-168
6' 0"	138-148	144-159	153-173

For girls between 18 and 25, subtract 1 pound for each year under 25.

Courtesy of the Metropolitan Life Insurance Company.

MEN

Height (with shoes on) 1-inch heels	Small Frame	Medium Frame	Large Frame
5' 2"	112-120	118-129	126-141
3"	115-123	121-133	129-144
4"	118-126	124-136	132-148
5"	121-129	127-139	135-152
6"	124-133	130-143	138-156
7"	128-137	134-147	142-161
8"	132-141	138-152	147-166
9"	136-145	142-156	151-170
10"	140-150	146-160	155-174
11"	144-154	150-165	159-179
6' 0"	148-158	154-170	164-184
1"	152-162	158-175	168-189
2"	156-167	162-180	173-194
3"	160-171	167-185	178-199
4"	164-175	172-190	182-204

Courtesy of the Metropolitan Life Insurance Company.

4

Vitamin E,
Wonder
of
the Ages

The latest vitamin recognized by the U.S. Government for its need in human nutrition is vitamin E.

Everything there is to know about this miracle "wonder of the ages" is in this chapter—culled from eminent doctors, health scientists, nutritionists, medical researchers, medical writers, and health journals and periodicals.

What doses? How often? Why?

You will learn how vitamin E can build your body's defenses against disease and help ward off illness, how it acts in your body, what may happen if you don't get enough, and how to tell when you need more.

I have been accumulating information over the years as to the unexpected extent of vitamin deficiency diseases, and I feel a definite moral obligation to pass this information on to such people as may be interested. The importance of these facts is clear in our vital statistics: "more people die from the end results of vitamin deficiency than from all other causes combined" (once we admit that heart disease and lowered resistance to infection come under this category).

The Most Powerful Weapon Against Disease

Of all the substances available to medical researchers, one of the most powerful weapons against disease is vitamin E. It is being used by many eminent medical specialists in dealing with heart and circulatory disorders, arthritis, diabetes, cancer, asthma, high blood pressure, emphysema, ulcers, anemia, colitis, varicose veins, sterility, mental retardation, and a host of other ailments.

A diabetic friend of mine was amazed to learn that studies show that among diabetics taking vitamin E for circulatory problems doctors noted a significant drop in insulin requirement.

Foods richest in vitamin E are wheat germ, corn oil, seeds, cottonseed oil, soybean oil, wheat germ oil, sunflower oil, liver, eggs, and nuts of all kinds.

Of course, vitamins alone can't and won't do everything for everybody, but they can do more than most people give them credit for. They can't harm you, in reasonable doses. They can relieve certain types of pain that you may think will never go away. They might improve the outlook of those suffering from emotional disorders and from heart trouble. They may be able, in short, to prevent or help a wide variety of ailments.

Mysterious Pains Yield to Vitamin E

Mysterious pains, suspected to be neuritic or arthritic in origin, are frequently suffered by persons beyond middle age.

This condition can be successfully treated with vitamin E concentrate.

Clinically, vitamin E concentrate has been found valuable in the treatment of sterility in both sexes. Probably the commonest indication of vitamin E deficiency is disappearance of the sex instinct, or its failure to appear at all. (The former situation is more common in the males and the latter in females. It should be understood that vitamin E is not a sex stimulant. In treating a condition of deficiency, its effect is merely that of renewing normality.

Vitamin E cooperates with vitamin A, not only in preventing sterility, but also in another function of vitamin A—the maintenance of normal epithelial metabolism. It is a useful aid in correcting conditions like eczema, urticaria, and dermatitis.

How to Protect
the Body Against Cancer

It is believed by less orthodox physicians that Vitamin E promotes the supply of magnesium and calcium to the tissues, helps to protect the body against cancer, and promotes the health of the sex organs.

The Non-Drug Answer
to Angina Pectoris

The pioneers in vitamin E therapy are Doctors Evan and Wilfred Shute, of the world-famous Shute Foundation in London, Ontario, Canada. The Shute brothers are best known for their work in treating cardiovascular disease, but the benefit of vitamin E in the veins is for all practical purposes identical to its action in the arteries. And as we have seen, a blod clot which tears loose from a vein in the leg is as dangerous as one in an artery and can easily bring about a heart attack. So the use of vitamin E for phlebitis is very intimately associated with its use in controlling heart disease.

Vitamin E is the non-drug answer to angina pectoris, according to Dr. Wilfred Shute. He's treated more than 30,000 patients for over 30 years with vitamin E and has achieved astonishing success—even though medical authorities, at least in public, avoid acknowledging his success.

Relieving Leg Pains

The Shute Clinic reports that vitamin E is very beneficial for circulatory troubles of the legs—varicose veins, Buerger's Disease, intermittent claudication, and leg cramps.

The Shute Clinic does not advise surgery for varicose veins as they end up exactly where they began after surgery. Some people have had several such operations, but they all end up the same way.

One of Dr. Shute's patients came to him after having suffered from varicose veins for a number of years. She had phlebitis in both legs and an acute thrombosis. There was also a swelling of feet and ankles and both legs had become badly discolored with "a dead heavy feeling in them."

She took 300 units of Vitamin E a day, and the aching disappeared after 6 weeks. But when she decreased her dose, her legs started to ache again. On 600 units a day her legs ceased to bother her at all, Dr. Shute reported.

Other Conditions
Treated with Vitamin E

A German physician reported that vitamin E lowered blood pressure in a group of 100 chronic hypertensives. He used 60 milligrams of vitamin E daily, reducing it gradually to 10.

Two West German physicians reported on many occasions that conditions helped by Vitamin E included sterility, premature births and stillbirths, recovery from abortion, lactation troubles, blood clots, angina pectoris, hardening of the arteries, ulcers, eczema, psoriasis, menopause, and disturbed menstruation.

What Vitamins Really Are

You might call vitamins "sparks" which are vital to the proper use of food for your body. Just suppose you had a stove or a furnace, all set up with oil or coal or gas, and you had NO match to light it. You could die of cold in spite of all the food in the world. Vitamins are like that. You can't have nutritional balance without them. Each of the essential vitamins performs a different and necessary function in your body; so you must get all the vitamins that have been recognized in human nutrition.

Why Vitamins Are So Important

It is interesting to note that in 1911 Dr. Casimir Funk discovered the first of the wonderful food factors to open the age of modern nutritional science. He called this "vitamin A." As other vitamin discoveries were made, they were called B, C, D, etc.

Let us see why vitamins ars so important. In the years throughout history, right up to our present century, men, women and children suffered with a variety of troubles which medical scientists now realize were caused by vitamin and mineral deficiences. For example, among early British sailors living on the high seas on a ration of salt pork, scurvy was a common illness. The problem completely disappeared when lime juice was added to the sailors' diet. (They've been called "Limeys" ever since.)

Over a hundred years passed before Nobel prize winner Dr. Albert Szent-Gyorgi discovered that the nutritional wonder ingredient found in limes and other natural fruits is vitamin C. Later research revealed problems which can come from vitamin deficiences, and the government, recognizing the nutritional value of vitamins, established daily vitamin requirements.

5

Vitamin C, the Miracle Medicine

It has been common knowledge for years that vitamin C (ascorbic acid) will prevent and cure a common cold. Nutritionists, doctors, researchers, and medical scientists have been telling you throughout the years to take large doses of vitamin C whenever a cold affects you.

It is about the only vitamin I know of that you can't take too much of, because the body will automatically eliminate the surplus.

Now, after years of experimentation, the latest findings are that vitamin C has been proven beneficial in many areas: from colds to allergies to arthritis to schizophrenia to diabetes to hay fever to cardiac conditions. According to neurosurgeon Dr. James Greenwood, Jr. of the Baylor University College of Medicine, vitamin C can also come to the aid of back, neck, or leg pain due to spinal disc injuries.

W. J. McCormick, M.D. of Toronto, Canada, goes so far as
to say that there is quite a bit evidence that a lack of vitamin C
might be one of the causes of cancer.

Every Part of the Body
Benefits from Vitamin C

The older we get, the more vitamin C we need. It protects
our health against viral and bacterial infections. It is helpful in
avoiding back surgery. It contributes to the health of the
arteries and is helpful to the health of the circulatory system.
Tests have shown that it can help to fight off many illnesses—
particularly heart disease, the number one killer. Studies have
shown that it can prevent advancing age. There is now evidence
that in massive doses it might indeed be the answer to cancer
therapy and prevention. Every part of the body benefits from
vitamin C.

One of the world's most distinguished scientists,
biochemist Linus Pauling, feels that, in addition to extending
life, vitamin C can reduce cancer, heart disease, and mental
disorder.

How to Avoid
Infections

If you are especially susceptible to infections, you may
need more of foods naturally rich in vitamin C than the rest of
us need. These foods include: all citrus fruit (including
oranges, grapefruit, lemons, limes, and tangerines), strawberries, broccoli, brussels sprouts, cabbage, guavas, kale, mustard
greens, green peppers, turnip greens, melons of all kinds, berries of all kinds, cauliflower, kohlrabi, tomatoes, fresh peas,
watercress, liver, and juices of all kinds.

There is evidence now that a vitamin C deficiency can lead
to some kinds of arthritis. Dr. A. P. Meikeljohn writes that it

has been found that arthritics have low counts of vitamin C in their blood. The recommended daily allowance of vitamin C for adults is from 55 to 60 milligrams.

It was reported in the July, 1973 issue of *Prevention* magazine that for some twenty years Dr. Klenner, an iconoclastic Southern doctor, waged virtually a one-man war against the Washington establishment with his radical views on vitamin C. He is convinced that massive doses of vitamin C are an absolute necessity in the body's struggle against the ravages of a whole host of illnesses ranging from pneumonia to burns to diabetes and even overdoses of barbiturates.

Dr. Klenner found that 60% of all diabetics could control their condition with diet and 10 grams of vitamin C daily. Even the other 40%, however, will need much less insulin and less medication overall if they follow this practice.

Death Takes a Holiday

Dr. Klenner says he has seen children dead in less than 2 hours after hospital admission, having received no treatment simply because the attending physicians were not impressed with their illness. A few grams of vitamin C given by needle while they waited for laboratory procedures or examinations would have saved their lives. In similar situations Dr. Klenner has routinely applied massive doses of vitamin C and consequently saw "death take a holiday."

Make sure that you are getting enough vitamin C, especially if there is a history of arthritis in your family. One cup of raw, green cabbage contains 50 milligrams of vitamin C, while one medium green pepper has about 125 milligrams.

According to Public Reports, about 17 percent of all Americans suffer from some form of arthritis. About 200,000 of these are below the age of 25. Rheumatoid arthritis afflicts about 5 million, with generalized symptoms that affect the entire body's joints, tissues around them, eyes, heart, and lungs.

Evidence of the value of vitamin C as a preventive of muscle stiffness comes from Dr. I. H. Syed, a London physician who wrote in the correspondence columns of the *British Medical Journal* that "muscle stiffness which arises after exercise or unaccustomed work can be prevented and treated by taking massive doses of vitamin C."

Dr. D. T. Quigley, in his vitamin chart (published by the Consolidated Book Publishers, Chicago), states that a deficiency of vitamin C results in, among other things, physical weakness, shortness of breath, rapid respiration, rapid heart action, and tendency to disease of the blood vessels and heart. Dr. Quigley also states that sudden death from heart disease in relatively young or middle-aged persons is caused, in a measure, by blood vessel and heart disease resulting from lack of sufficient foods containing vitamin C.

Dr. Robert Cathcart III of Nevada, an orthopedic surgeon, has successfully treated over 5000 patients for viral diseases with massive doses of vitamin C. He believes that any viral disease can be conquered by large doses of vitamin C—and the sicker you are the more vitamin C you require. Most of the foods rich in vitamin C—such as melons, citrus fruits, broccoli, and tomatoes—are summertime favorites. Therefore, it is important to take a vitamin C supplement daily in the winter, especially if you are afflicted with a common ailment.

A letter to the *British Medical Journal* reports the experience of a Canadian doctor who treated a patient suffering from schizophrenia with one gram of vitamin C every hour for 48 hours—a gigantic dose not to be taken without a doctor's supervision. At the end of that time she was mentally well. She was discharged from the hospital and remained in good mental health.

A Dramatic Response to
Malignant Cancer When Radiation
and Drugs Were Delayed

Dr. Irwin Stone tells us that Dr. Dean Burk and his group at NCI published in the scientific journal *Oneology* (oneology is the study of cells) a description of their findings that vitamin C kills cancer cells and is at the same time harmless to normal cells. Dr. Stone describes a case of malignant lymphoma (cancer) in a truck driver who was treated by Dr. Ewan Cameron. The vitamin C treatment was begun only because the orthodox treatment with radiation and drugs was delayed and the man was deteriorating rapidly. He was given 10,000 milligrams a day by mouth.

The response was so dramatic that the patient said he felt quite well, his appetite returned, his night sweats stopped, and he had a general sense of well being. His enlarged liver and spleen returned to normal size and other symptoms of the disease subsided. He went back to work taking 10,000 milligrams of vitamin C daily.

For some unknown reason, the patient stopped taking the vitamin and one month later was back in the clinic with recurring symptoms. The usual dose of vitamin C failed to bring improvement. The disease progressed. He was then given 20,000 milligrams per day, intravenously, for two weeks, and 12,500 milligrams daily by mouth thereafter. "A slow and sustained clinical improvement was shown and examination about six months later showed him to be normal in all respects" says Stone. The patient went back to work and continued to take this large amount of vitamin C every day with no evidence of active disease.

Complete Remission of Leukemia

Dr. Stone tells us that *Medical Tribune* printed a case history in which doses of up to 42,000 milligrams of vitamin C were given to a victim of myelogenous leukemia. The result was complete remission of the disease. Every time the vitamin dosage was experimentally stopped the symptoms returned. But within six hours after the vitamin dosage was started again, the patient improved and remission recurred. "You would think," says Stone, "that someone in these many years would have tried this harmless megascorbic therapy in the thousands of cases of leukemia that appear each year. A search of the (medical) literature has failed to reveal anyone publishing a check on these exciting clinical results."

How Cancer Patients Are Living Four Years Longer Than Expected

Cancer researchers have been very lax in testing vitamin C. But one physician in Scotland has discovered that his terminal cancer patients were living four years longer than expected and in reasonably good health when he gave them massive doses of vitamin C. NCI scientists have given healthy subjects vitamin C for a few days and have found that it stimulates the body's defense systems, usually increasing immunity.

The consequences of vitamin C deficiency are as follows:

1. Scurvy symptoms—ranging from severe to mild degrees. The symptoms include skin hemorrhages (due to weakened capillaries), pyorrhoea, loose teeth, decalcification of bones, and susceptibility to dental caries.

2. Impaired adrenal (and thyroid) function, with consequent cardiac and vascular disease.

3. Anemia due to impaired iron metabolism.

4. Stomach and duodinal ulcers. (Vitamin C is essential to the normal secretion of gastric mucin.)

5. Diseases of blood vessels and capillaries (fragility, hemorrhages, tendency to bruise easily, "black and blue spots," purpura hemorrhagicia, varicosities).

6. Diseases of gums (hemorrhages, sore gums, pyorrhoea).

7. Tooth degeneration (necrosis, caries).

8. Joint and bone changes (decalcification, friability).

9. Mucus membrane hemorrhages.

10. Destruction of bone marrow.

11. Tendency to epithelial lesions (ulcerations of mouth, intestine, etc.).

12. Increased susceptibility or reduced resistance to infections.

13. Retarded growth and loss of weight.

14. Physical weakness, depression, and irritability.

15. Rapid respiration and heart action.

16. Blood degeneration (tendency to certain types of anemia, reduced hemoglobin, destruction of bone marrow).

17. Development of heart weakness.

18. Increased weight and enlargement of spleen, liver, stomach, intestines, and kidneys.

19. Atrophy or hypertrophy of glands:

    (a) Reduced secretion of adrenals.

    (b) Morbid secretion of thyroid (toxic goiter).

20. Development of arthritis (rheumatic tendency).

21. Development of edematous conditions.

22. Tendency to raised temperature.
23. Complications of pregnancy and lactation as well as ill effects to new born (abortions).
24. Possible sterility.
25. Lowered glucose tolerance.
26. Cataract.
27. Predisposition to allergic conditions.
28. Scurvy.
29. Death.

Today we are beginning to see the light as to the biochemical reactions that are behind these symptoms. We know that vitamin C is a diffuser and distributor of calcium to the tissues and the blood. It is undoubtedly in the later years of life that the consequences of vitamin C deficiency become more apparent.

Apparent functions of vitamin C:

1. Essential to health and integrity of endothelial tissues (raises resistance to infections).
2. Essential to proper development of teeth.
3. Essential to oxygen metabolism.
4. Regeneration of blood cells.
5. Maintains proper blood-clotting time.
6. Tendency to structural tissue changes.

Vitamin C deficiency, through a reduction of calcium ions, can deaden the sympathetic stimulus to the arteriole musculature, which is normally necessary to maintain dilation. This interferes with the blood supply to certain organs or extremities, such as in certain forms of arthritis.

Enter Laughing:
An Enigma of the First Magnitude

In a booklet published by *Prevention*, the chapter "Give Me the Marx Brothers, Give Me Vitamin C" describes the most astonishing case history I have ever come across of complete recovery from a crippling disease. It is truly the "miracle of miracles."

Norman Cousins, former editor in chief of *Saturday Review*, was hit by debilitating illness after his return from a particularly stressful stay in Russia. According to *Prevention*, he ached all over and within a week had difficulty moving his neck, arms, legs, and even his fingers. His jaws were almost locked. Hospitalized, he lay in bed in agony. His chances for recovery were one in 500.

Cousins recounts his struggle and ultimate recovery in *The New England Journal of Medicine* (December 23, 1976). The blood sedimentation rate is often elevated during infection, inflammatory disease, and cancer. Cousins' was extremely high. Generally, the normal rate is between zero and 20. A rate of 80 is considered decidedly abnormal. Cousins' rate shot up to 115—certainly nothing to laugh about. His condition was diagnosed as ankylosing spondylitis, a progressive disease of the joints of the spine primarily affecting men.

Cousins took a lively interest in every aspect of his illness and treatment, searched the medical literature—including *Prevention*—for insights, clues, and guidance, and, with a big assist from massive doses of vitamin C, laughed his way out of a crippling disease which doctors believed to be irreversible. I have never known of a man with such quiet perseverance, fortitude, courage, and will power—and in the midst of excruciating pain. This, to me, is an enigma of the first magnitude, so "miraculous" it almost defies belief!

6

Vitamin A,
the Amazing
Health Rejuvenator

Another important vitamin is vitamin A. It is necessary for normal vision, promotes growth, builds resistance against infection, and is helpful in warding off the ravages of old age because of its influence on the glands. Research has shown that vitamin A also protects the body from stone formation and helps to maintain alkalinity. It prevents kidney stones and bladder and gall stones.

Foods high in vitamin A are cabbage, carrots, egg yolk, celery, prunes, oranges, parsley, spinach, kale, tomatoes, eggs, butter, cheese, and liver.

Protection from Infection

The action of vitamin A is principally upon the epithelial surfaces, the skin and the mucous membranes; in fact all of the lining surfaces from mouth to anus. It protects us from infection at every point through which germs might enter the body.

Stomach ulcers, infections of the intestinal tract, colitis, or ulcerations in any part of the intestinal tract all show a lack of vitamin A.

Vitamin A is definitely helpful in warding off the ravages of age, because in some fashion or another it protects the body from stone formation. Research has shown that vitamin A increases the life span because of its influence on the glands.

Vitamin A may be found useful in treating the following conditions: (1) Lack of appetite in undernourished children. (2) Lowered resistance of the epithelium to bacterial invasion and epithelial irritability. This includes such otherwise diverse conditions as susceptibility to colds, gastritis, cystitis, and nephritis. Of course, there are other factors causing disease, but when vitamin A deficiency is present disease tends to persist and does not respond to conventional therapeutic measures. Albuminuria without apparent cause, especially in children, is often controllable with one capsule a day of vitamin A. Acute cystitis is often immediately controlled; so are certain types of gastritis. (3) Certain individuals have found that an occasional vitamin A capsule maintains a normal bowel function. As yet, we have no theory to offer, except that vitamin A is known to be essential to liver function. (4) Dropsy where there is present liver dysfunction. It must be remembered that vitamin A is essential to kidney function as well as the function of the liver, and its value in this situation may be attributable to the beneficial action on each organ. (5) Stones or gravel in the kidney or bladder can be considered a definite result of vitamin A deficiency. The accompanying susceptibility to infection is a serious matter. The calculi tend to become abscessed, and the only rational treatment (besides surgical removal) is a high vitamin diet and vitamin concentrates. Two capsules of vitamin A, daily, produce definite results.

Vitamin A is formed in the body from carotene, the coloring material in butter, yellow vegetables, and cereals. It is also obtained from eggs, liver, carrots, and the green leaf vegetables.

How to Avoid Jaundice

Carotene in a purified form is widely sold as vitamin A. This should not be considered an effective source. It is my opinion that most persons who have a deficiency of vitamin A have for some reason lost their ability to convert the carotene into the vitamin. In certain countries where the diet is confined to vegetables high in carotene (squash as an example), some persons, presumably those who have lost the conversion power, become yellow in color, simulating jaundice, differing only in that the whites of the eyes are not affected.

It is my prediction that some other dietary factor as yet unidentified will be found to be necessary for this conversion. Meanwhile, I suggest vitamin A to those who are sufficiently critical to expect a definite clinical result in each case where its use is indicated.

The specific action of vitamin A that relates to infections is its ability to insure an epithelial integrity that will prevent the mechanical entrance of germs. Colds and influenza are believed to be caused by a filterable virus; so the ability of vitamin A to protect against the entrance of effective agents may be of little or no value in those particular infectious diseases.

Vitamin A deficiency in test animals, however, is particularly effective in reducing the resistance to pus germs—with resulting infections of sinuses, tonsils, mastoid, etc. Here we have visible microorganisms to deal with, and not a filterable virus that can penetrate openings too small to admit germs that can be seen in the microscope.

Why a Shortage of Vitamin A
Caused the Influenza
Epidemic During World War I

It is more than probable that a widespread reduction in the supply of vitamin A such as occurred during the First World War (mainly because of butter substitutes) was the basic reason for the influenza epidemic that spread over the entire civilized world. The paucity of other high vitamin foods and the atttendant low intake of all vitamins, no doubt, were aggravating factors. Infective agents are known as a general rule to increase in virulence in proportion to the lack of opposition by the normal defensive factors. A person with low resistance may develop a severe attack of influenza, for instance, and thereby infect another subject who normally would resist the disease and fail to contract it from a person suffering from a less virulent form. That is how epidemics get under way.

The severity of the cold and influenza epidemics has caused some observers to suggest that possibly the general irradiation of milk may be responsible, because of its destruction of vitamin A. There is no doubt that the practice of irradiating foods indiscriminately has become more or less a commercial racket.

Enhancing the Body's
Defenses Against Cancer

Vitamin A is necessary for healthy skin, and since it is important for the eyes, extreme deficiency results in irreversible blindness. It will deplete rapidly during stress and very likely aggravate the incidence of ulcers. Stress can also lead to other diseases.

A daily spoonful of cod liver oil, rich in vitamin A, could cure rickets. Robert Rodale, of *Prevention,* says that "Recent research has indicated that Vitamin A can enhance the body's defenses against invaders as common as respiratory infections and as deadly as cancer."

A spokesman for the National Cancer Institute said that vitamin A and its synthetic analogs have been successfully used to prevent cancer of the skin, lung, bladder, and breast in experimental animals.

Michael B. Sporn, M.D. of the National Cancer Institute, writes in *Nutrition Reviews* that such experiments have been conducted in regard to cancer of the trachea (windpipe), the bronchus (those branches of the windpipe that enter the lungs), the uterine cervix, the stomach, and the vagina. Dr. Sporn explains that the data at hand clearly indicate that no human population at risk for development of cancer should be allowed to remain in a vitamin A deficient state. Considering the relatively trivial cost of supplementation of the diet with a minimum daily requirement of vitamin A, this is certainly a goal which should be met for the entire population.

Vitamin A, in emulsified form, has been used in conjunction with Laetrile in the biological treatment of cancer in Germany, the country that leads the world in cancer weapons.

Dr. Max Odens of London indicates that vitamin A seems to prevent cancer of the lung.

Some Complete Cancer Remissions

A series of 20 patients suffering from various head, neck, and tongue cancers was treated exclusively with vitamin A emulsion at the Janker Clinic and Hospital in Germany. There were no failures and some complete remissions.

In over 100,000 patients treated with larger doses of emulsified vitamin A, side effects have been tolerable and fully reversible.

Possible results of vitamin A deficiency:

1. Retarded appetite, growth, and development (due to interference with assimilation).
2. Disturbed dental and bone development (atrophy).
3. Susceptibility to infections as well as slow healing of reticuloendothelioma and epithelium, due to degenerative change in structures of skin and mucosa.
4. Presence (due to lowered resistance) of infections of eye (corneal ulcers) and degeneration of eyes, night blindness, total blindness, infections of the ear, infections of genitourinary tract, infections of mucous tract (tonsilitis), infections of respiratory tract (pneumonia, tuberculosis), infections of gastrointestinal tract (diarrhea), infections of sinuses.
5. Interference with successful reproduction and lactation (loss of sex impulse), sterility in the female by failure of ovulation or resorption of fetus, sterility in the male by temporary injury to seminiferous epithelium, prolonged gestation, retained and diseased placenta, difficult delivery.
6. Development of pernicious anemia, secondary anemia, rickets, gastritis, bronchitis, kidney and bladder disorders and renal dysfunction, formation of stones, nephritis, cystitis.
7. Atrophy of organs and glands (testes, liver, spleen, thyroid, pituitary and salivary).
8. Degenerative skeletal muscle lesions develop.
9. Ophthalmia, conjunctivitis.
10. Acne, which occurs more often during adolescence.
11. Development of psoriasis, ulcers, goitre, thyroid.
12. Cancer of the lung.

The American Cancer Society recommends chemotherapy, radiation, and surgery as treatments for cancer. The dietary pathway to prevention and cure has been largely ignored by orthodox medicine. But according to recent research on the effect of vitamin A on cancer and precancerous conditions, this vitamin should be given top priority.

Vitamin A Discovered in 1915

Vitamin A was discovered in 1915 by McCullum and Davis. They found that certain laboratory animals which were deprived of certain foods, such as butter and other animal fats, developed an eye disease and eye infection which eventually led to blindness. They found that an animal which had definitely developed the eye disease might, in cases where the disease had not progressed too far, be cured by restoring the proper food. The food investigations showed that the protective element which they were studying existed in certain fruits, yellow colored vegetables, and the green leaves of vegetables.

They found that not only would eye diseases develop where this substance was lacking in diet, but also that certain other parts of the body became diseased, and the character of the disease in these cases was found to be in the nature of an infection. This work proved that food plays a major part in protecting certain parts of the animal body against the more common infections.

The animals on the deficiency diets suffered invasion of certain organs and tissues by low grade micro-organisms. The structures in which low grade infections had occurred were the eyes, the tonsils, and other lymphatic structures, and the sinuses connected with the nasal cavity (antrums, ethmoid cells, frontal sinuses, mastoids, sphenoids, etc.).

In the animals that were killed and examined after such an experimental diet deficiency, abscesses were found in the sinuses and tonsils, and in some animals there were also collections of pus in the ear and mastoid cells.

Action to Take
Against Infections

Vitamin A is considered one of the main elements of protection, in a basic manner, against all infections. It undoubtedly has a decided effect in protecting against the infections which cause ordinary colds, and which localize in the nasal cavity, the throat, and the respiratory tract.

The body has the power of storing vitamin A to a considerable extent for future needs. An abundant supply of it in early life safeguards the body against later infection as well as providing for present needs. This does not mean, however, that the need of vitamin A is confined to the young. An amount sufficient to support normal growth and health may still be insufficient for the added demands of reproduction and lactation and for resisting the infections more common in early adult life. Long-time feeding experiments conducted on rats have shown increasing benefits throughout succeeding generations in the continued use of liberal amounts of vitamin A.

Vitamin A, in its acid form, is considered to be the best therapy for acne, in view of the troubles one must go through to obtain a cure. It is to be applied directly to the skin. Because of its irritant effects, vitamin A cannot be tolerated by everyone. There is a great possibility that acne may return, usually within three to six weeks if the application of vitamin A is stopped.

Dr. John D. Straumfjord, originator of the treatment, said that oral vitamin A supplements may keep acne away, once the condition is cleared up and the acid applications are discontinued.

More Than Vitamin A Needed

Dr. Merlin Maynard of San Jose, California, reported on the successful treatment of acne using vitamin D and calcium. In addition to receiving vitamin D and calcium, Dr. Maynard's patients followed a special diet of lean meats, fresh fruits, and green vegetables with no sweets, chocolate, pastries, or greasy or highly seasoned foods or carbonated drinks.

Vitamin A, derived from fish liver oils, aids in the growth and repair of body tissues and helps maintain healthy skin. Aside from the maintenance of good eyesight, it builds strong bones and teeth, and forms rich blood.

It also has been indicated in medical circles that vitamin C plays an important part in controlling acne. Practically all medicated cosmetics are harmful to acne, when the cause is actually internal and not merely a surface condition.

Effective Psoriasis Therapy

Psoriasis appears to be a family trait, and is not contagious. Any part of the body may be afflicted with it, but strangely enough, not the face. Psoriasis most commonly afflicts the scalp.

Dr. Phillip Frost and Dr. Gerald D. Weinstein, both of the Department of Dermatology, University of Miami School of Medicine, discovered that vitamin A, in its acid form, brought remarkable relief from the itching and unsightliness of psoriasis in 24 out of 26 patients, and these effects were noticeable after only a week's treatment. Halibut liver oil is an excellent source of vitamin A. It is considered advisable to limit intake to less than 50,000 units of vitamin A daily.

How to Get Better Results

The use of B vitamins in treating psoriasis cannot be overlooked. Dr. John F. Madden, a physician in St. Paul, Minnesota, has achieved positive results in treating psoriasis with vitamin B-1 (thiamine), an ointment, and a low fat diet. Some physicians have reported good results with vitamin B-12. Proper diet is very important to sufferers of psoriasis. They should avoid meat and dairy fats. Lecithin supplements should be a staple in their diet.

Action to Overcome Bronchitis

Cigarette smoking and polluted air are the leading causes of bronchitis. Vitamin A and vitamin C manage to give us a significant measure of protection.

Dr. Richard W. Stone, Medical Director of the New York Telephone Company, blamed this increasing level of pollution for the high incidence of chronic respiratory disease. The Metropolitan Life Insurance Company has found that chronic respiratory ailments such as bronchitis are 33% more common among holders of its industrial policies, who breathe polluted factory air on a daily basis.

A London physician, Dr. Max Odens, conducted a long term clinical study, based on the knowledge that vitamin A is involved in the maintenance of a healthy mucous membrane lining of the respiratory tract. Other physicians have obtained miraculous results by eliminating milk from their patient's diet. Medical science does not offer any cure for bronchitis. Giving up tobacco and fortifying yourself with a highly nutritious diet will enable nature to help.

A New Era

Since we are now in an era where doctors, medical scientists, researchers, nutritionists, and medical writers are continuing to come forth rapidly with the latest in the use of vitamins, therapies, and supplements for the treatment of disease, one must make a special effort to keep abreast of the new developments and their significance.

The "Nine-Day Inner Cleansing and Blood Wash for Renewed Youthfulness and Health" was discovered by me in 1947 when not too much was known about vitamins, minerals, and supplements. It is accountable for the continued good health I have been in all those years. I have not had to resort to drugs with their serious side effects.

Today the world around us is reverberating with the latest therapeutic discoveries and new world shaking theories. If employed these will tend to increase the effectiveness of the Nine-Day regimen. "Healing the body *first*" is its chief object.

Leading doctors are irrationally and illogically extreme in their opinion and practice of attacking the disease first.

While on the subject of the Nine-Day regimen, I must stress the fact that it is not a crash diet, nor is it a diet in the true sense of the word. It is a "natural" and harmless therapy of cleansing the body of poisonous wastes (toxins) and foreign matter that have been stored up and accumulated around the intestinal wall since childhood, causing disease.

7

Continued Developments
in the Struggle
for
Good Health

In recent years there have been a number of dramatic discoveries about the effect of food elements, such as vitamins, and other non-drug therapies, against even the most dreaded diseases. Harold E. Buttram, M.D., has informed me of several of these. Dr. Buttram recently spent some time at the Janker Clinic and Hospital in Bonn, Germany—probably the most successful hospital and clinic for the treatment of cancer.

Evidently Europe is much ahead of the United States in acceptance of unusual methods of cancer treatment. Dr. Buttram reports that after billions of dollars being spent on the war on cancer in the United States, the occurrence rate and death rate are little changed from what they were twenty years ago.

The orthodox treatments with chemotherapy, radiation, and surgery alone are evidently not doing an adequate job.

Presently, there is a growing wave of public opinion calling for a very basic re-evaluation of these types of treatment. The benefits of these customary medical therapy methods are coming under increasing question and doubt.

Recently, an official of the American Cancer Society stated that there has been no dramatic reduction in the rate of death from breast cancer in the past four decades. At a recent conference on environmental carcinogenesis in Houston, sponsored by the American Cancer Institute, American Cancer Society, and other organizations, the statement was made that current medical treatment in this country has had little impact on the death rate from cancer.

Hardin Jones, recognized as an authority in medical statistics, has stated that survival rates for cancer patients have not improved during the era of chemotherapy and radiation, with the exception of childhood leukemia and Hodgkins disease.

An "Exodus" of Patients

In recent years, we have witnessed a mass "exodus" of cancer patients from the United States to foreign countries, particularly to Germany, for alternate therapies which are illegal or unavailable here. Within the United States, for good or ill, there has evolved an underground railroad for cancer patients, in some respects reminiscent of the underground railroad during the days of slavery for escaped slaves seeking freedom.

It should be explained that two distinct and separate approaches in cancer therapy are emerging:

1. Standard or orthodox medical therapy, based largely on the use of toxic-type drugs, radiation, and surgery.

2. Biological therapy directed at the building or stimulating of the body's own immune systems and

resistance against cancer, the restoring of normal and healthy body organ functions, and the cleansing from the body of carcinogenic toxins.

In both of his visits to several treatment centers in Germany, Dr. Buttram witnessed something better in the form of biological therapy.

Striking Improvements Reported

Dr. Karl Hansberger of Munich has reported on three thousand women with mastectomies for breast cancer. His report showed 84% improvement in three year survival for those women who were placed on biological therapy, an astounding improvement over the current statistics available for those cases not receiving biological therapy in conjunction with surgery, radiation and chemotherapy.

In an interim report sent to the German Ministry of Health, Dr. Hoefer and Dr. Sheef, the heads of the Janker Hospital and Clinic, stated: "In several cases we were able to bring tumors the size of baby's head, which were beyond any further therapy by cytostatics and radiation, to a complete remission."

In Dr. Buttram's own tour of the Janker Hospital and Clinic, two random cases stand out in his mind. One was a breast cancer with an ulcerated tumor the size of a small orange brought into complete remission using isophosphamide with radiation. Another was a cancer of the lung, the size of a small orange, which disappeared completely on chest x-ray several weeks following isophosphamide.

Confidence in Licking Cancer

Motion picture and TV star Fred MacMurray fought cancer of the throat with "Laetrile" method and diet which includes no meat, or very little, lots of fish, and carrot juice twice a day with a little cream in it. Emulsified vitamin A is used in conjunction with Laetrile, which is a substance derived from pits of apricot and peach pits.

Complete Remission of Cancer

Here is another interesting case history worthy of mention: Robert Fontaine, age 63, suffered from cancer of the nasal passages and double vision. After 3 weeks of treatment with Laetrile and a strict diet at the Centro Mexico Del Mar, A.P. in Mexico, he was discharged from the hospital with complete remission.

A Natural Agent for
the Prevention of Cancer

The "Nine-Day Inner Cleansing and Blood Wash for Renewed Youthfulness and Health," if employed once a year, should prevent you from contracting cancer by a thorough cleansing of your insides of an accumulation of poisonous wastes and foreign matter. If this stored matter is allowed to stagnate, the result might be a debilitating disease.

No Harmful Side Effects

It is sometimes said that Laetrile produces harmful side effects. Yet the wife of Red Buttons, motion picture and TV star, has been taking Laetrile treatments in West Germany for five years, since she suffers from cancer of the lymph glands. The star was quoted as saying she has taken these treatments without any side effects at all. Dr. Hans Nieper, her physician, used methods nobody in the United States had heard about. In the U.S., doctor after doctor had said there was no chance; they had given her up to die. It is reported that Red Buttons is so vehement about all this that he has said, "Every time I read about Laetrile being a hoax, I swear to God, I think I'm living in Nazi Germany."

An Open Letter
to Senator Kennedy

Dr. Buttram was so concerned about the son of Senator Edward Kennedy having lost a leg to cancer that he sent an "open letter" to the senator urging him to order an independent investigation by Congress of the merits of unorthodox medical care. He urged Senator Kennedy to hear from medical men such as John Richardson, M.D., of California, and Paul Wedel, M.D., of Oregon, doctors who have been involved in Laetrile therapy for many years and have had a wealth of clinical experience with Laetrile and other related therapies.

Dr. Buttram pointed out that today public opinion is calling for a very basic re-evaluation of cancer therapy in the United States. In spite of the fact that many billions of dollars have been poured into cancer research, the benefits of the customary methods of medical therapy are coming under increasing question and doubt. Dr. Buttram urged Senator Edward Kennedy, as a public servant, to select an important group of medical experts and send them to foreign countries such as Austria and Germany where they are achieving superior results in terms of survival rates of cancer patients with the use of biological therapies. He also suggested that Senator Kennedy go and survey work being done with Laetrile at cancer centers such as the Janker Clinic and Hospital at Bonn, Germany, where they have developed four of the most potent anti-cancer agents known to man.

Pyridoxine,
the Precious B-6 Vitamin

Another important disease-fighting element is vitamin B-6, found in many common foods. Now we have startling new information linking lack of pyridoxine (vitamin B-6) with three of the most pernicious diseases of modern times—diabetes, hardening of the arteries, and chronic liver disease.

Low levels of vitamin B-6 seem to disturb the activity of insulin, which is the body's regulator of blood sugar.

Lancet (March 19, 1977) printed an article by two Cambridge University pathologists about the possible part played by vitamin B-6 in the development of hardening of the arteries. Drs C. I. Levene and J. C. Murray tell us that a certain enzyme is responsible for the health of the body substances collagen and elastin, which, joined together, make up the inner lining of arteries. There is now strong evidence that pyridoxine is involved along with the enzymes in this linking process, so that enough of this vitamin must be present for the lining of the arteries to be healthy.

Pregnant women are commonly deficient in vitamin B-6. It is suggested that all pregnant women be given adequate vitamin B-6.

Foods High in Vitamin B-6

In food, vitamin B-6 is available in liver, blackstrap molasses, brewer's yeast, wheat germ, canned tomatoes, soy beans, brown rice, and a number of other nutritious foods.

Pyridoxine, like other B vitamins, is harmless. Any amount of it which is not needed by the body will be excreted harmlessly.

Nutrition Reviews (June, 1977) reviewed the relation of

the B vitamin pyridoxine to chronic liver disease. It was found that alcoholism was a pernicious cause of liver disease, but this condition was helped by vitamin B-6.

Good-bye to Cholesterol Scares

The 20 year era of blaming cholesterol diets for heart disease and other ailments is now in question. A Scandinavian study shows that cholesterol in food is not to be blamed for high cholesterol levels in blood.

We are now being told by responsible investigators that the more high density fats there are in the blood the *less* chance there is of having a heart attack. However, Dr. George V. Mann, D.M.D. of Vanderbilt University, says that fats double the incidence of gallstones.

Drugs that lower the levels of cholesterol in blood have been found to be ineffective in preventing deaths from heart attacks. According to Dr. Mann, there is no safe and efficacious drug known for the management of cholesteremia (high blood cholesterol).

Degenerative Diseases Rare in China

If we want to convince ourselves that the American diet is terribly deficient, all we need to do is compare it with the diet of the average Chinese. In China there is practically no arthritis or diabetes, and other degenerative diseases are relatively rare.

The basic diet in China consists of rice, soy bean cakes made from soy bean milk, fresh green vegetables, and fish. It is better from a vitamin standpoint than our meals loaded with white flour, white sugar, cold-storage meat, pasteurized milk, and butter and cheese made from the same pasteurized milk.

No Variation in the
Chinese Daily Diet

The Orientals do not butter or sugar the rice they eat. There is practically no variation in their daily diet since every meal every day is the same. They eat about a pound of rice a day, which cooks up into three very large bowls. Thus, they are avoiding foods that are overly-rich in animal fats and sugar which constitute a great part of the American diet. Semi-brown rice is available. But for some reason, maybe taste or even as a status symbol, most Chinese prefer white rice. There is a low number of fat Chinese, very low compared to the U.S.

The Medical Melon
of the Tropics

Papaya offers properties not found in any other fruit or vegetable. The U.S. Department of Agriculture reports: "It is well recognized that the papaya contains peculiar and valuable digestive properties which make it of great value in the diet." It is known as the medical melon of the tropics.

Papaya is a luscious melon shaped fruit that grows in clusters on short palm trees. It grows only in the tropics where the natives have valued it as both food and medicine for centuries. As the fruit ripens, the skin turns from green to an orange-yellow, and the sweet juicy fruit becomes a deep yellow. The smooth flesh contains very little fibre, and its aroma and flavor are delicately tropical and delicious. The papaya is frequently referred to as the "Medicine Tree" because nearly every part of the plant contains some medical properties.

An Amazing Powerhouse
of Natural Nutrients

Brewer's Yeast is a fantastic source of natural nutrients— packed by Nature with food energy. The cells contain vitamin

B-1, vitamin B-2, iron, vitamin B-12, vitamin B-6, protein, all the amino acids, and phosphorus.

For thousands of years, yeast has been used in baking, wine making and brewing, and it has been discovered to be a valuable food on its own. Each tiny brewers yeast cell is rich in protein (just like human body cells) and contains an amazing powerhouse of natural vitamins, minerals, carbohydrates, enzymes and *all* the essential amino acids.

The Lowering of High Blood Sugar

Brewer's yeast lowers high blood sugar and cholesterol levels. Chromium and a mysterious substance called the Glucose Tolerance Factor may eventually solve many of the health problems associated with diabetes and pre-diabetes. These two substances—both available in brewer's yeast—can also reduce cholesterol and triglyceride levels.

High, low, and variable blood sugar are known to have been regulated with chromium and the Glucose Tolerance Factor (GTF). They help to keep blood sugar levels where they should be.

The best sources of chromium and other helpful trace minerals are brewer's yeast, bran, whole grains, seeds, nuts, liver, and meat.

Most Americans are chromium deficient, largely because we eat foods from which chromium has been removed by refining. Troubles with blood sugar usually occur among older people. A chromium supplement of 150 micrograms has been successful in regulating blood sugar levels in older people and those who had become diabetic after middle age.

Roughage Is Important to Health

Scientists now believe that "high fibre," or "roughage," is important to health. Fibre is the "woody" or cellulose part of foods. Digestion is helped by high fibre foods because fibre is the ingredient that helps to move foods through your intestines. One of the best dietary fibres is bran, which comes from the outer husks of wheat kernels. This valuable fibre actually absorbs moisture and helps smooth the movement of your foods.

Dozens of magazine articles and medical journal reports indicate that the lack of fibre in our daily food may be one of the important reasons for many health problems. The "civilized" food we eat—which has much less fibre than the rough simple foods of "primitive" peoples—causes us to suffer from far more digestive ills, overweight, and other diseases of civilization. Fibre content is missing from most of our foods because they are processed.

Tremendous Food Value
in Sunflower Seeds

Sunflower seeds have 22 vitamins, minerals, and protein in every single kernel. They are Nature's own ready-packed vitamin and mineral storehouse, according to *Coronet* magazine, which states that "The Sunflower seed boasts significant quantities of thiamine, niacin, and Vitamin D. It is so rich in iron that few foods, other than egg yolks and liver, can compete with it." The protein content of sunflower seeds is even higher, per pound, than the protein in meat. And the protein in sunflower seeds is easily digested and highly nutritious. They contain many other valuable elements: calcium, phosphorus, iron, vitamin B-1, vitamin B-2, iodine, and vitamin D. And they are also rich in poly-unsaturated oil.

Sunflower seeds were being cultivated by the Indians before Columbus arrived. Today, Russia is the world's largest producer of sunflower seeds. Only now are Americans learning the tremendous food value of these unusual seeds. Our scientists are discovering that sunflower seeds are superior in many ways to all other seeds and grains.

A Sustaining Food

Carob, from the Middle East, is the source of the wondrous beans the Bible called "manna from heaven." Theologians believe that this is the food which sustained St. John the Baptist in the wilderness, and that is why it is called "St. John's Bread." For those who cannot eat chocolate, carob is a gift from heaven. It looks like chocolate, tastes like chocolate, and is just as satisfying to eat.

Our Gift from the Seas

Kelp, an edible seaweed, is extremely rich in iodine, and iron, calcium, potassium, chlorine, sodium, sulphur, magnesium, and phosphorus. It is an excellent source of vitamin E and vitamin A, and a good source of vitamin B; it also contains vitamin D.

Robert Rodale, in his booklet *The Prevention System for Better Health*, writes that "Kelp is our Gift from the Seas." Rodale also notes that kelp may well become the good food of the future; the elements in kelp may keep our diets sufficiently stocked; it is clean seafood; it grows as fast as two feet each day; it matures too rapidly to absorb much pollution; and it takes from the water only the life-giving nutrients it needs to support such rapid growth. Few plants can match the wealth of essential minerals in kelp. Studies have shown that kelp derivatives can inhibit the body's absorption of certain poisonous substances.

Mr. Rodale makes a fitting observation: "Ever since one of our Stone Age ancestors enjoyed his first bite of seaweed, the sea has been the great provider of good foods."

The Foundation of Any Diet, Designed to Reduce Cholesterol Levels

Lecithin balances bile composition. Taken every day in generous amounts, it will protect you against gallstones. It consists largely of poly-unsaturated fatty acids, the foundation of any diet designed to reduce cholesterol levels. It prevents fats from clumping together.

Lecithin is usually extracted from soybeans and is found in egg yolk, salmon roe, calf liver, and yeast. The egg yolk is the greatest source.

Little-Known Health Ideas

Over the years, I have made the following observations about health and long life. Check these for yourself. Do you know that:

- Only two percent of all heart attacks occur during exercise; most of them occur during rest, and fifty percent during sleep.
- Worry kills more people than work.
- You can die of a broken heart.
- Asparagus has cured many cancers.
- Diabetes is a deadly disease you can live with.
- Spinach juice, about one pint daily, has often corrected the most aggravating case of constipation in a short period of time.
- An enema of a quart of buttermilk and blackstrap molasses will alleviate the symptoms of colitis.
- Brewer's yeast, high in iron, normalizes blood sugar and is considered to be an almost complete food.

- Magnesium is a natural safeguard against kidney stones.
- Coffee and spinach are harmful for arthritis sufferers.
- We are digging our graves with can openers.
- Blackstrap molasses has cured malignant cancers, growths of the uterus, ulcers, and growths of the breast.
- Laetrile is the most powerful and useful anti-cancer agent known to man.
- Honey is the best food for the heart.
- Black radish juice is known to dissolve gallstones.
- Formaldehyde, which is used as a spray on frozen vegetables to keep their color, is harmful to health.
- The cardboard kind of supermarket tomatoes are not ripened. They are gassed in order to keep them red.
- Cancer strikes one out of every four Americans.
- Too much salt early in life can set the stage for high blood pressure in later years.
- Daily use of fresh apple cider vinegar and water will slim you down without dieting or the use of drugs.
- Vitamin B-12 is beneficial for bursitis.
- Diarrhea can be overcome in no time.
- Overweight people complicate almost any disease they contract.
- Germany leads the world in cancer weapons.
- Blackstrap molasses, gram for gram, contains more iron than any other food except brewer's yeast.
- Honey contains practically all of the vitamins and is a most effective remedy for shortness of breath.
- Mae West, famous motion picture star of the early thir-

ties, takes an enema every day and fasts three days a month. She's 85 years young.

- Heart attacks by young people who do not have a heart condition are becoming increasingly common because of neglect of daily elimination.
- Acute indigestion has put many a businessman in the obituary column long before his time.
- Carrots are excellent for diabetics.
- Honey is a most effective remedy for chronic fatigue.
- Garlic is an aid in high blood pressure.
- Spices like pepper, cinnamon, and cloves are aphrodisiacs. They give much needed zest to the sex organs.
- Kelp and vitamin A are playing important parts in the treatment of bronchial asthma.
- Vitamin E helps to protect the body against cancer, and promotes the health of the sex organs.
- Papaya is a very nutritious juice. It contains properties not found in any other fruit or vegetable.
- Brewer's yeast lowers high blood sugar and cholesterol levels.
- Only now are Americans learning the tremendous food value of sunflower seeds.
- Kelp, our gift from the seas, is an edible seaweed, extremely rich in iodine, iron, and calcium.
- The latest findings are that vitamin C has proven beneficial in many areas from colds to allergies to arthritis to schizophrenia to diabetes to hay fever to cardiac conditions.

I must stress the importance of the foregoing observations on health because they are the ones most often overlooked.

8

Living a Clean and Healthful Life

One hundred or more years ago, before the advent of modern industrialization and commercialism, it was a simple matter in this country to live a clean and healthful life. Pure spring water was available in many areas. Air was not polluted to any extent. There still remained vast forest areas which perpetually cleansed and renewed the air by utilizing carbon dioxide and releasing oxygen. Even in urban areas, the average person had far more exercise than today, for lack of modern conveniences if for no other reason. The soils were generally virgin and fertile, and foods themselves were as yet untouched by commercialism. Americans in those days were, on the whole, a hardy and rugged people.

Processed Foods, Synthetic Drugs and Chemicals in Vogue Today

In contrast to those former conditions of innocence, we now have almost universal pollution involving every phase of the human environment. In addition to air and water pollution, there are literally thousands of synthetic chemicals being added to commercial food products, almost all of which are foreign to the biological systems of life. The foods themselves are seldom left in their life and health building states. They are adulterated, denatured, and devitalized by various forms of processing.

Although our present medical system has made great advances, particularly in control of infectious diseases, reduction of infant mortality, and advances in surgery, it is nevertheless a system based largely on the use of synthetic drugs and chemicals. To all intents and purposes, America has become a drug-oriented and drug-dependent nation.

Unprecedented Blood Pollution

In a manner of speaking, it would not be far amiss to say that we are living in an era of unprecedented blood pollution, the consequences of which are as yet only dimly realized. A rather strange phenomenon of our time is the fact that the public in general seems to be more aware and aroused concerning the dangers of these problems than the scientific and professional communities.

80 to 90% of Cancer
Environmentally Caused

If there are dangers from foreign chemicals and adulterated foods, what is the nature of these dangers? We do know that there has been a steady increase in chronic diseases including cancer in recent decades. In a recent conference held in Houston, Texas, under the sponsorship of The American Cancer Society, National Cancer Institute, and other organizations, it was estimated that 80 to 90% of cancers are environmentally caused. We also know that we are witnessing a virtual epidemic of nervous/mental disorders with related problems including crime, juvenile delinquency, sexual perversions, broken homes, and various types of addictions.

Eminent Religious Devotees Are Pioneers of Nutrition

During the first half of the 20th century, there were a few far-seeing nutritional pioneers such as J. I. Rodale, founder of *Prevention*, Weston Price, R. S. Clymer, and Roger Williams who warned about the total impact of environmental pollution, synthetic drugs and chemicals, and denatured foods, not only on the physical health of the individual but on the mind, nervous system, and the personality. Especially unique among these early workers was Dr. R. S. Clymer, who served both as a practicing physician and a minister in a church of Christian denomination. Because of his dual role, he emphasized—perhaps more than any others—the dangers not only to physical health but also to the mind, personality, *and spiritual welfare* of the individual resulting from environmental pollution, commercialization of the food industries, and almost total dependence on the use of drugs within our present medical system. Dr. Clymer was the founder of the Clymer Health Clinic and Complex in Quakertown, Pennsylvania.

Religious people of many faiths consider it a duty to live a clean and healthful life. At least for those religiously inclined, it is reasonable to assume that *any substance with adverse effects on the mind and personality may also adversely affect the spiritual welfare of the individual.* A vast literature exists on this particular topic, but a few representative studies of the past and present may suffice for our present purposes.

Astounding Health of the Hunzas

In the early 1900's a British surgeon, Dr. Robert McCarrison, was stationed in northern India where he became interested in the astounding health and physiques of the local tribe of people, the Hunzas. Among these people he commonly found individuals living past the age of 100 years—and some of these individuals had even retained their teeth without cavities. Cancer, heart disease, and other chronic diseases were virtually unknown.

After years of study and observation, McCarrison performed experiments on albino rats in which he placed one group on a diet basic to the Hunzas, largely consisting of fruits, vegetables, and dairy products. To another group of rats he fed a diet which was common to the poorer classes of England at that time (also very similar to diets among teenagers in the U.S. today) including white bread, sweetened tea, boiled vegetables, jams, and tinned meats.

Among those rats fed the Hunza diet, Dr. McCarrison reported simply that disease was abolished. In the first 2 years of the experiment there were no illnesses and no deaths in the adult stock, and except for several accidental deaths, no infant mortality. These rats were very tame, and they were easily made into pets.

In the second group of rats, deaths were frequent, and disease was universal. Furthermore, the rats developed what Dr. McCarrison referred to as a rat neurasthenia. They were nervous and apt to bite their attendants; they lived unhappily together; and by the 16th day of the experiment they began to kill and eat the weaker ones amongst them.

Raw vs. Cooked

In 1946 Francis Pottenger reported a series of studies done on 900 cats over a ten year period in which he placed one group on a diet of *raw* meat, *raw* milk, and cod liver oil. This group reportedly had good resistance to vermin, parasites, and infection. Abortion was uncommon, and mother cats nursed their young in a normal manner. Their organic development was complete, and they functioned normally.

The second group of cats was fed *cooked* meat, milk, and cod liver oil. Abortion among these cats was common, running about 25% in the first generation and 70% in the second. Many cats died in labor. Disease was universal, and by the third generation the kittens were so degenerated that none survived 6 months, thereby terminating the strain.

Concerning behavioral changes noted during the experiments, cats that were fed cooked meat were reported as irritable. Females were dangerous to handle, sometimes viciously biting the keeper. The males were more docile, often to the point of being unaggressive. Sex interest was slack or perverted, and in second generation cats there was a tendency to reversal in physical characteristics, the males becoming more effeminate in body configuration and the females more masculine.

Relationship Between Sugar and Alcoholism

In demonstrating the relationship between sugar and alcholism, Dr. Roger Williams, former president of the American Chemical Society, did a simple experiment with rats in which he gave one group of rats sugar as their source of carbohydrates. To a second group he provided potatoes. To both groups of rats he made available plain water and alcoholic beverages in separate containers. Those rats provided the potatoes drank only water while those given sugar rapidly became addicted to alcohol.

Mental Illnesses Brought
About by Sugar Intake

A great deal has been written by such renowned authors as Carlton Fredericks, J. I. Rodale, founder of "Prevention," Paavo Airola, and E. M. Abrahamson concerning the interrelationship between sugar intake and mental illness and criminality. These works have been very popular in the health literature and need no recounting here.

The development of interest in a relationship between chemical food additives and personality changes has been quite recent, and has largely been due to the work of Dr. Ben Feingold as a pediatric allergist at the Kaiser Permanente Medical Center in San Francisco. Again, this work has been well reviewed in the health literature and is familiar to most readers. Very briefly, Dr. Feingold has shown strong evidence that there is a causal relationship between artificial food colorings and flavorings and the development of personality changes, including hyperactivity in children.

Loss of Memory and Coordination
from Chemical Food Additives

In the text, *Mental and Elemental Nutrients* by Carl Pfeiffer, M.D., the relationship between copper and lead toxicities and hyperactivity in children is reviewed.

Actually, at a much earlier time, Dr. R. S. Clymer was one of the first to report observation of mental deterioration resulting from chemical food additives—with entire personality changes, rapid loss of memory, and loss of coordination.

The very great potential of drugs for alteration or control of the personality was reviewed in a startling article in *Fortune* magazine (March 1977) entitled "A Preview of the Choose Your Mood Society."

In this article the author, Gene Bylinsky, reports that drug technology is moving along so fast these days that chemical behavior modification may soon be a reality. One scientist reported to the author that there is a developing potential for nearly total control of human emotional status, mental functioning, and will to act. As a final statement in the article, the author quoted Joel Elkes, a pioneer biochemcial psychiatrist, in the following comment:

> This field poses the ethical dilemma of science at its most poignant. The specter of a drug-polluted or drugged society is here to stay, until faced responsibly through a process of education and gradual permeation by an enlightened regulatory process.

Whether one agrees with it or not, the natural health movement is rapidly emerging as a significant force in our society, a force which continues to grow and thrive in spite of, at times, ruthless opposition. Within this movement, one finds large numbers of individuals and families seeking to gain or maintain health by pure water, unpolluted environment, simple and vital foods, and often by the use of biological and drugless methods for care of health problems. Some have estimated that this element may constitute as much as 10% of our population at the present time.

As stated earlier in this article, any person who has had much experience in working with this group of people will probably agree that many, perhaps a majority, are attempting to follow more natural health practices as part of their religious and moral beliefs. Governmental interference and intervention in these practices constitutes just as much a violation of religious freedom as if the police were to invade our churches, lock the doors, and prevent worship.

Although there are few formal doctrines in modern churches concerning today's natural health movement, the fol-

lowing scriptural verse is often quoted in health literature as a
reference:

> And God said, behold I have given you every
> herb bearing seed, which is upon the face of the earth,
> and every tree, in which is the fruit of a tree yielding
> seed, to you it shall be for meat.
>
> Genesis 1:29

Our present law makers and legislatures appear to be
largely oblivious to the real nature of this question. Americans
generally are patient people, sometimes gullible; but
historically they have always stood firm on principles, *especially* in times of crisis. The time has come when rational and
equitable answers must be found, restoring rights originally intended by the U.S. Constitution.

The Bill of Rights

As the story goes, Dr. Benjamin Rush, one of the signers of
the Declaration of Independence, proposed that health
freedom be added to the Bill of Rights as one of the guaranteed
rights under the Constitution. His proposal was voted down,
not because of any disagreement, but because the existing Bill
of Rights was thought to be adequate in guaranteeing health
freedom as inherent within the other specified freedoms, especially religious freedom. Benjamin Rush stated:

> The Constitution of this Republic should make
> provision for healing freedom as well as religious
> freedom. To restrict the art of healing to one class of
> men and deny equal privileges to others will
> constitute the bastile of medical science. Such
> restrictions are fragments of monarchy and have no
> place in a Republic.

In these days of expanding government controls with bureaucratic regulation and intervention in the private lives of American citizens, it is becoming increasingly clear that health freedom and religious freedom are inseparable. If one is lost, the other is equally forfeited.

Although at times these laws may appear stern, they are in connection with today's rapidly growing "natural health movement," the religious undertones are clearly evident to those who have had experience in working with this group of people. An analysis will reveal three common denominators in our modern natural health movement and the religious or moral principles found in many of our churches.

First, almost all individuals religiously inclined have at least some degree of feeling and appreciation for nature and nature's laws as part of God's creation. If the world was created by God, it follows that nature's laws *are* God's laws.

Although at times these laws may appear stern, they are constantly working for our welfare and benefit. It is precisely this feeling or sentiment that is almost universally found in the natural health movement with its emphasis on "natural foods" and "natural healing."

The Concept of Blood Pollution

The second common denominator has to do with the concept of "blood pollution." This concept was very simply and beautifully expressed by Dr. Harold Buttram in an article in *Let's Live Magazine*, June 1975. This was one of a series of articles reviewing major religions of the world from a standpoint of dietary practices. Quoting from the article:

> There were other instructions that reinforced a belief, common to most religions, that the spirit of God will not dwell in an unclean tabernacle deliberately polluted by the person himself.

Always implied within this concept is the conviction that foreign or unclean substances, whether in the form of chemicals, food additives, unnecessary drugs, or unclean or devitalized foods, can affect an individual adversely, not only physically but also mentally, morally, and spiritually. This undoubtedly explains the great extremes sometimes seen in those trying to avoid chemicals, foods, etc. considered unclean or foreign to the human system.

One of the most forceful statements ever made on this subject is found in the writings of Dr. R. S. Clymer, considered by many to have been one of the foremost pioneers in the nutritional field. Dr. Clymer stated:

> Destroy a man's mind, his reasoning ability, his imagination, and neither gold, silver, mansions, freedom, love, or anything else will matter to him. This is easily accomplished, is being accomplished by simple means: the creation of disease in his body by *toxic substances in his food;* shattering his nervous system, hardening his muscles, and deteriorating his mind; making of man, the godly human, a sub-human creature, a lesser animal, a vegetation, souless.

Individual Responsibility Concerning Matters of Health

Finally, the third common denominator has to do with the principle of individual responsibility concerning matters of health. While doctors and hospitals are often necessary in care of sickness and injuries, health can be maintained only by individual effort, reasonable self discipline, personal cleanliness and hygiene, and daily application of the laws of health.

We Are Living in a "Synthetic" Period

Without a doubt, today's natural health movement is a reaction to the times in which we live. If we had to choose a single word to characterize our present period, the word "synthetic" would be one of the most appropriate. This would undoubtedly be true for any phase of our complicated society, but it is probably most true for our present medical system and methods of health care. Although this system is humane in purpose, and although it has made great advances for human welfare in many respects, it is nevertheless a system based largely on the use of drugs and chemicals entirely foreign to the biological system of the human body. This in itself would be well and good if individual patients were allowed freedom of choice in seeking alternate methods of care when desired. What is wrong is the fact that patients do not have free choice in seeking alternate methods of care for many types of health problems. Medical doctors for their part are commonly faced with ostracism by their colleagues, separation from medical societies, or worse whenever they deviate from the rigid confines of orthodoxy. This is especially reprehensible when one considers that many of these patients as well as doctors are motivated in their actions by moral or religious principles.

Many parallels can be drawn between present conditions and those which existed in 16th century Italy during the life and times of Galileo.

It will be recalled that modern science had its first beginnings during the Italian Renaissance between the 14th and 17th centuries. Scientists in those days were definitely the underdogs, so to speak, having to cope with the combined forces of church dogma, superstition, and profound ignorance. Certainly, this was true in the case of Galileo. It was then generally believed that the earth was the center of the universe and that the sun, moon, and stars rotated about the earth. When Galileo proposed that the days and nights were due to rotations of the earth itself, there was a storm of protest from church officials. Ultimately, he was delivered to the inquisition because of his heretical teachings. In those days the church establishments had absolute political power, and any challenge to church dogma was considered treasonable, often resulting in imprisonment or death.

Today in America many feel that we are witnessing the emergence of a somewhat comparable situation, but with the positions reversed. Now the scientific institutions, through government bureaus such as the F.D.A. and H.E.W., carry political powers on much the same scale as church institutions in earlier times. Policies dictated by these bureaus are made with very little recognition of the moral and religious beliefs of American citizens, as these beliefs apply to matters of health.

Within our present health system, many Americans are compelled by law to conform to health programs and medical care which are alien to moral or religious beliefs. Conversely, they are deprived by law of those types of health care that they would prefer if granted free choice. Dare we say it? It is a bad situation when honest and moral people in our so-called free country are compelled by law to violate moral and religious principles.

Ultimately, the struggle for health freedom can be won only through true scientific research, because all things having to do with health care must be proven by rigorous and objective testing. However, it is precisely in the realm of research that we have the roots of our problem.

Why Our System Is Disease and Drug Oriented

Our medical system as it exists today is basically disease oriented and drug oriented. The concept of health, health for its own sake, is largely foreign to medical thinking. There is unfortunately little reverence or even recognition of innate healing forces within the human body, much less an interest in study of nutritional or biological methods to enhance these healing forces.

Within governmental bureaucracy today in the field of health care, we find an impenetrable ban on any meaningful research dealing with alternate, unorthodox, biological, or nutritional approaches to health care—a ban no less inflexible than that encountered by Galileo in his struggles for scientific freedom. In Galileo's time, those who challenged established dogmas of the period were called heretics. Today they are called "unscientific quacks." The terms are different, but the spirit of intolerance is the same.

9

Improving Health
Through
Food Chemistry

From the earliest records that we have, fasting has at all times been regarded as essential to health and longevity by all the nations of antiquity. And by the more religiously inclined it has been considered a very necessary adjunct to spiritual enfoldment.

The Egyptians were considered to be the healthiest and longest lived people of any of the nations of antiquity, and it was an invariable habit among them to fast during the first three days of the new moon and in place of food to take purgatives. In the Hebrew records, we find that Moses fasted for forty days on two different occasions. We also are told that it was the custom and practice of Elijah, Daniel, Isaiah, and all other prophets to fast. Almost all religions teach fasting of some kind. Therefore, we can understand why Jesus took it for granted that anybody aspiring to spiritual power should fast. He gave no commandment because it was generally understood that any serious minded person would adopt this course. He said, "When ye fast, be not as the hypocrites are." In his famous interview with Nicodemus he very clearly announced the Law when he said, "Except one be born of water and the Spirit (Air), he cannot enter into the kingdom of God." This means that the change of consciousness from the purely physical and mental to the spiritual comes about only when man has won the complete victory and has become master over the organs and faculties of his mind. No one can ever have a consciousness of spiritual power to any great degree until he knows what it is to be totally free from every desire of the flesh—for at least a period of time. That is to say, he must learn by actual experience to substitute water and breathing for the more substantial forms of food.

Why the Body Must Be Healed and Not the Disease

Every sick person has a more or less mucus-clogged system, such mucus being derived from the undigested and un-eliminated, unnatural food substances accumulated from childhood on. Disease is an effort of the body to eliminate the waste and toxins. It is the body that must be healed and not the disease. The body must be cleansed and freed from waste and foreign matter. This cleansing cannot be accomplished in a few days, as compensation must be made for the wrong commited against the body for a period of many years. The process of cleansing and healing the body must be systematic and gradual.

The human organism is an elastic pipe system through which liquids and gases circulate. The digestive tract is the largest tube in the body, and it is here that the denser food substances enter the body to be broken down and chemically organized into blood and other vital saps that nourish the body.

It is in the digestive tract that clogging and constipation begin. The diet of civilization is never entirely digested and the resultant waste entirely eliminated. This causes the entire pipe system of the body to become slowly congested and clogged, beginning with the digestive tract, extending into the arteries and veins, and finally reaching the finest openings in the capillaries and skin pores gradually clogging even the cells themselves. The beginning of every disease can be traced to the intestinal tract and to the food consumed. Knowing this to be a scientific fact, let us then intelligently search for the means that will help to eliminate the stored up waste and bring about a normal and natural function, thus restoring the body to its natural state of strength and radiant health.

Nature's Law of Compensation Against Every Disease

Fasting has been known for hundreds of years as nature's only infallible law of compensation against every disease that the human body is subject to. We read in Genesis that fruits and herbs are the food for man, but man has gone far from the path he started on, and we can all testify to the suffering he has gone through. Even in this enlightened age disease and premature death take tremendous toll of human lives. It is high time that we begin to learn the right way of living.

Air is the power that keeps you alive, for without air you cannot live ten minutes. Therefore, we know that breathing and the right kind of elimination will change sickness into health and sorrow into happiness.

Why Deep Breathing Is Vital

We often hear people say, "I have no vitality." Just what vitality is, no one seems to know. Vitality is that tremendous power which creates a higher and superior state of health. Vitality is Breath. Have you ever seen a flat chested individual who had much vitality? No. The individual who has great vitality is *always* breathing deeply, and has a good chest development. Now we know that breath is vitality, and in order to have vitality we have to breathe, and breathe, and then breathe some more.

The Beginning of Disease

When the intake of food into the body is greater than its normal requirement, the excess has to be eliminated through the various organs of elimination, stored up as fat or waste, causing congestion and interfering with normal functions of the body. This is the beginning of disease. The individual becomes the unsanitary receptacle of his own waste products, which often become dissolved into fine solutions and find their way into the circulation, poisoning the blood, and penetrating every cell of the body. This causes deposits in the organs that are least able to throw them off and eliminate them from the system.

Every pain that racks the flesh is the voice of Nature saying, unload, purify! With purification comes peace. If you want health, happiness, or spiritual understanding, then clean your body inside, and while you are house-cleaning, go to the upper chamber and clean out the mind. With a clean mind and a clean body, all good things are possible.

How Right Living
Brings Health

You can eat your way into paradise physically, but you cannot pass the gate watched over by the angel with the flaming sword until you have gone through the cleansing fire of fasting and diet. There are those who long to possess the very last gift that life can hand them, but they do not, and will not work for it. They want health, wealth, love, and spiritual attainment, but do not want to earn it. Life gives you all that you earn, but no more. When we look at our body, distorted, out of shape, old, and ugly, it is not pleasant to think that we have just what we earned. But it is a pleasant thought that by right eating, right breathing, and right thinking we can earn and have a beautiful body, and we know that no one can take it from us but our own selves. It is a very comforting thought to realize that we create our own conditions through the Law of Cause and Effect. Wrong living produces disease, and right living brings health. So let us learn to live the New Way and hear the voice of our higher-self saying, "Well done my good and faithful servant, enter here and now into your reward of perfect health, greater capacity for enjoyment, clearer mental vision, and true spiritual development."

A Warning to Clean Up

Some will say, "I have tried to fast and it made me sick." True, as soon as you stop eating, the elimination begins to take place. The longer you go without food, the more waste matter is thrown into the blood stream which carries it to the various organs of elimination. While this waste matter remains in the blood we become sick. This should be a warning to clean up, but is it? No, we add more food, stop elimination, and continue adding more waste to the already encumbered body with its ten to thirty pounds of stored up waste matter. We excuse ourselves saying, "I can't fast." Oh, you doubtful man, you Peter of little faith, who are moved by each wind and sink easily! The time is coming when man will be ashamed to admit sickness. It will mean the same thing as saying, "I have violated the law; my temple is unclean."

"Ye Suffer from Yourselves;
None Other Binds You That You Bloat and Die"

Hardly one person in a hundred is true to the type Nature intended him to be. We all might be the image and likeness of God, if we had the spiritual backbone and knowledge enough to take ourselves in hand. No sight is to be more deplored than the great flesh-pots who call themselves men and women, who are not so at all; they are simply walking sanitary vats, into which appetite and self-indulgence have turned too big a stream of waste material. Hospitals and sanitariums are full of this overfed unpurified lot. They are a menace to the world. They are sending out thoughts of sickness, talking sickness, and filling others with the evil of wrong living. Their only desire is to be rid of the effects of their ignorance, but not of the ignorance itself. Try to dislodge their little god of appetite, and see how they will defend him. Tell them to fast, breathe, and change their thinking, and they turn away disappointed. One cannot help but think, "Ye suffer from yourselves; none other binds you that you bloat and die." But there are many who are truly seekers, only waiting to find a way, and to those I say, "There is only one way, eliminate, cleanse, and be free."

Disease: The Cure Is the
Opposite of the Cause

Have you ever stopped to think what the lack of appetite means when you are sick? Or how animals overcome illness in spite of the fact that they have no doctors, no drug stores, and no machinery to heal them? Nature shows us there is only one disease, and that one is caused through eating. Every disease, whatever name man gives it, has only one cause and one remedy. The cause is improper eating. The remedy is the direct opposite: first, give the body a complete fast, and second, feed it correctly afterwards.

A New Way of Fasting

Most people cannot stand a real fast at first. Their bodies are filled with waste matter, and as soon as they stop eating these poisons are absorbed into the blood stream, causing much discomfort and even pain. Let me explain what goes in the body during a fast. We know that the body is a machine, made of rubber-like material, which has been over-expanded during many years of wrong eating. Therefore, the functioning of the organism is obstructed by unnatural pressure of clogged tissues against the blood stream. As soon as one stops eating, this pressure is rapidly relieved: the avenues of circulation contract and the blood becomes more concentrated as superfluous water is eliminated. This goes on for a day or two, and you may even feel better than before. But the obstruction of the circulation increases because the blood meets with resistance from sticky mucus that has been pressed out from the inside walls of the organs. This may cause pains and aches in the organs most affected. The blood stream must overcome, dissolve, and carry with itself mucus and poisons for elimination through kidneys, skin, and other organs of elimination.

When you fast, you eliminate the primary obstructions of wrong eating. This results in your feeling relatively good, or even better than when eating. But as I have already explained, you bring new secondary obstructions from your own waste in the circulation and you eventually feel miserable. You—and every one else—blame the lack of food. If you will notice the urine after a day of fasting during which you have felt miserable, you will no doubt find small strings of mucus. Then you can see for yourself what has been taking place and why you felt so bad. Fasting serves two purposes: first, it relieves the body from obstructions of solid unnatural food; and second, it is a mechanical process of elimination that contracts tissues and presses out mucus that is causing friction and obstruction in the circulation. As long as the waste is in the circulation, you will feel miserable during a fast. The cleaner the body is, the longer you can fast. But in the old way of water fasting all this cleansing work was done by and with the original old blood composition of the patient—and there are few people who can stand the result of their own wrong eating all at once.

As we have eaten our way out of health, let us now eat our way back. By experimenting, and through trial and error, I have developed a pleasurable *new way* of fasting to replace the miserable old fashioned way of fasting that allows nothing but water. Now you won't mind fasting at all.

Fasting for longer periods than 3 days should be under professional supervision. I have chosen seven days for a fasting period, to be taken every 6 months. You will benefit by it healthwise from the intake of fresh fruit and vegetable juices selected. These vegetables have dissolving properties and high chemical content. You will also take an "Elimination Broth." Here is the recipe:

> 2 cups of celery
> 2 cups of carrots
> 1 cup of spinach
> 1/2 cup parsley

Grind through a food grinder, saving the juices. Add one quart of water and simmer for 15 to 20 minutes. Strain and serve hot.

After the fast, your body will be much cleaner than it was seven days ago. You will have more strength and will not tire as easily. Your body will be ready to be remade. What is most important is that you will actually have gone through the rigors of fasting in a most pleasurable way. The fresh fruit and vegetable juices are sustaining and prevent weakness. Here is your seven-day fast:

FIRST DAY

Upon rising in the morning: juice of one lemon in a glass of hot or cold water without sweetening.

Breakfast: A glassful of fresh orange juice. A glassful of fresh grapefruit juice, 2 hours later.

Luncheon: Elimination Broth, hot. A glassful of cranberry juice, 2 hours later.

Dinner: Elimination Broth, hot. A glassful of papaya juice.

SECOND DAY

Upon rising in the morning: juice of one lemon in a glass of hot or cold water without sweetening.

Breakfast: A glassful of fresh orange juice. A glassful of fresh grapefruit juice, 2 hours later.

Luncheon: Elimination Broth, hot. A glassful of apple juice, 2 hours later.

Dinner: Elimination Broth, hot. A glassful of fresh grape juice, unsweetened.

THIRD DAY

Upon rising in the morning: juice of one lemon in a glass of hot or cold water without sweetening.

Breakfast: A glassful of fresh orange juice. A glassful of fresh grapefruit juice, 2 hours later.

Luncheon: Bowl of hot fresh tomato juice. A glassful of fresh pineapple juice, unsweetened, 2 hours later.

Dinner: Elimination Broth, hot. Juice of one fresh lemon in a glass of water, 2 hours later.

FOURTH DAY

Upon rising in the morning: juice of one lemon in a glass of hot or cold water without sweetening.

Breakfast: A glassful of fresh orange juice. A glassful of fresh grapefruit juice, 2 hours later.

Luncheon: Elimination Broth, or hot fresh tomato juice.

Dinner: Elimination Broth. A glassful of fresh pineappe juice.

How do you feel? If your body is very toxic, you are feeling miserable and are ready to quit, blaming the diet for your distress and discomfort. Your body is dissolving mucus and toxic matter faster than it can be eliminated, or neutralized. Re-read the foregoing pages and resolve to stay on the diet for the next three days. Your reward will be well worth the trouble.

FIFTH DAY

Upon rising in the morning: juice of one lemon in a glass of hot or cold water without sweetening.

Breakfast: Dish of fresh berries, fresh peaches or melons.

Orange or grapefruit juice between meals, if desired.

Luncheon: A glassful of pure apple juice. A glassful of cranberry juice, 2 hours later.

Dinner: Elimination Broth, hot. A glassful of grape juice, unsweetened.

SIXTH DAY

Upon rising in the morning: a glassful of unsweetened pineapple juice.

Breakfast: A glassful of fresh orange juice. A glassful of fresh grapefruit juice, 2 hours later.

Luncheon: A glassful of pure apple juice. A glassful of papaya juice, 2 hours later.

Dinner: Elimination Broth, hot.

SEVENTH DAY

Drink as much fresh fruit juices as you desire the whole day.

Always remember to take an herbal laxative each night during this period of elimination to assist the process of cleansing.

A New Outlook on Life

Now you have gained a new outlook on life, and you have added many years to your life. But that is not all. You have a cleaner body than you had seven days ago. You have more strength and do not tire so easily. Your body is ready to be remade—and as all things are built according to the image held in the mind, now is the time to create youth and beauty in this new body.

Here are the rules to be carefully followed while on this elimination treatment:

- Clean the intestines every day.
- Take deep breathing exercises every morning and evening, or whenever convenient during the day.
- Get into the fresh air and sunshine as much as possible.
- Rest in bed as much as you can. Do not over-exert or undergo undue strain.
- Take warm baths before retiring: cleanse the skin with mild soap, then take a 15 minute bath in half a tub of warm water to which 1 ½ pounds of Epsom Salts have been added. This will open and cleanse the pores of the skin and induce elimination during sleep.
- Keep your vision on a new body, for we build the thing we visualize.

Here is something I want you to read over and over, until you cannot forget it: *Elimination can only take place when the stomach is empty of food.* It is during the period of rest and sleep that the cells and organs release poisonous waste. It can readily be seen how little time the body has to accomplish this when we consider that the average person eats three meals a day, and some people even eat before going to bed. Now you can see how necessary it is to have *long periods* between meals. No day is long enough for three meals. No one needs a meal the first thing in the morning. A glassful of orange juice, grapefruit juice, tomato juice, or some fresh fruit is sufficient. If you employ this every other morning, you will add years to your life's enjoyment by this one habit alone.

God Doesn't Dwell
in an Unclean Temple

Remember this: The cleaner the machine is, the smoother it runs and the more power it has. A dirty machine never works well. Your body is a very wonderful instrument, made up of the minerals and chemicals of the earth and air, and it is loaned to you while you are here. Your contract reads that as long as you keep it in good condition, you can stay in it, for God doesn't dwell in an unclean or broken temple. As long as your body is chemically perfect, you have the power to attract every good thing to yourself.

You cannot extract life from a dead substance. So how can you expect to put life into your body by eating dead food? Learn to eat live food. Anything that you have to kill before you can eat it is not a good food for you. In fact, all the foods which have to be cooked and fried for a long time and then seasoned before they are fit to eat are not the ideal foods for man.

Always bear in mind that *raw food is live food*, and to be healthy one must have a certain quantity of it every day.

The Body Is Yours to Mold

So far, I have talked about the physical body and what you can do with it when it is in good repair. In other words, you have been cleaning house, and now that you have every corner clean, you will find that you have many things you had forgotten about—things you have not used before in this body, but still have stored in the sub-conscious mind, ready to come forth as soon as the body is in tune. Our mind for the first time becomes conscious of higher laws. We find that a new energy flows through our body, and we feel that life is the greatest gift and blessing that could be given to us; in fact, we have connected ourselves through a clean body with life. We put off the old body of limitations and in its place we build with new materials a new and durable body, perfect in its strength, harmony, and beauty. As we know that all things are created by thought, so the first thing we must do is to change the mental plate. We have a new picture—a new blueprint to build our body by. We are going into the upper chamber to clean out the mind, and as we have eliminated the waste and poison from the physical to give shape and form to our body, so likewise we clean the rubbish from our mind and replace it with a perfect picture.

The mind is the master, the thought is its tool, and the body the plastic material. It is yours to mold, fashion, and design according to the pattern held in mind. Therefore, make your picture beautiful and perfect and work toward that end.

The elimination program given alone will benefit you most if repeated once every three months the first year and every six months thereafter until you have rejuvenated and rebuilt your body to your satisfaction. Remember that years of wrong living have caused much damage; so don't be discouraged if a complete change is not accomplished in a single elimination period. Repeat it again and again, until you have accomplished the desired result. Should you experience unpleasant symptoms during the elimination period, such as headache, nausea, and pains in different part of the body, do not be alarmed. You are drinking only 100% live juices which cannot cause you any harm. (But *remember*: Fasting for more than 3 days should be done under professional supervision.) You will feel so much better when the elimination is over that you will not mind the temporary inconvenience.

Foods and Their
Chemical Elements

POTASSIUM	CALCIUM	IRON
Tomato	Watercress	Sorrel
Kale	Dill	Lettuce
Rhubarb	Kale	Spinach
Lettuce	Turnips	Leek
Turnip	Cabbage	Rice
Sorrel	Lettuce	Strawberries
Dandelion	Dandelion	Radishes
Celery	Swiss Chard	Asparagus
Rutabaga	Spinach	Parsley
Cabbage	Romaine	Liver
Swiss Chard	Okra	Bone Marrow
Watercress	Leek Leaf	Kohlrabi
Cucumber	Radishes	Romaine
Cauliflower	Skim Milk	Swiss Chard
Beets	Celery	Cabbage
Radishes	Cottage Cheese	Onions
Leek Leaf	Buttermilk	Pumpkin
Eggplant	Turnips	Artichoke
Lima Beans	Goat's Milk	Watermelon
Parsnip	Lemons	Rhubarb
Mushroom	Tomatoes	Celery
String Beans	Cow's Milk	Rutabaga
Spinach	Chives	Oysters
Brussels Sprouts	Rhubarb	Cucumbers
Kohlrabi	Strawberries	Gooseberries
Dill	Blackberries	Tomato
Limes	Cranberries	Kale
Potato Skin	Orange	Turnips
Artichoke	Cucumbers	Beets
Carrots	Carrots	Dandelion
Soya Beans	Asparagus	Horseradish
Molasses	Onions	Mushrooms
Kidney Beans	Sea Fish	Dill
Skim Milk	Whole Grains	Cauliflower
Turnips	Beechnut	Prunes

POTASSIUM

Asparagus
Peaches
Apricots
Grapes
Prunes
Watermelon
Onions
Bitter Herbs
Sweet Potatoes
Cherries
Lemons
Huckleberries

MAGNESIUM

Chick Peas
Tomato
Spinach
Lettuce
Dill
Dandelion
Wheat Germ
Rice
Sorrel
Watercress
Cabbage
Romaine
Beets
Kale
Celery
Whole Oats
Rutabaga
Kohlrabi
Turnips
Blackberries
Swiss Chard
Apples
Almonds
Barley (whole)

CALCIUM

String Beans
Pumpkin
Peas
Dates

PHOSPHORUS

Kale
Radishes
Wheat Bran
Rice
Pumpkin
Mushrooms
Buttermilk
Goat's Milk
Sorrel
Cucumbers
Dill
Brussels Sprouts
Romaine
Swiss Chard
Cauliflower
Cabbage
Spinach
Turnips
Rhubarb
Soya Beans
Barley (whole)
Lettuce
Celery
Cottage Cheese
Egg Yolk
Beans
Peas
Oats (whole)
Almonds
Walnuts
Currants
Asparagus

IRON

Raisins
Potato Skin
Black Figs
Beef
Carrots
Cherries

SULPHUR

Kale
Watercress
Brussels Sprouts
Mustard Greens
Horseradish
Cabbage
Egg Yolk
Cranberries
String Beans
Spinach
Sorrel
Turnips
Raspberries (red)
Cauliflower
Radishes
Dill, Chive
Onions
Garlic
Lettuce
Cucumbers
Parsnip
Peas (green)
Figs
Tomato

SILICON

Lettuce
Asparagus
Horseradish

MAGNESIUM

Rye (whole)
Orange
Lemons
Grapefruit
Chive
Onions
Sea-Fish

FLUORINE

Cod Liver Oil
Goat's Milk
Mackerel
Roquefort Cheese
Swiss Cheese
Oysters
Oxtail Broth
Gelatine

CHLORINE

Tomato
Celery
Lettuce
Goat's Cheese
Spinach
Dill
Egg White
Butter
Whey
Cabbage
Kale
Parsnips
Beets
Turnips
Cucumbers
Carrots
Swiss Chard
Watercress

PHOSPHORUS

Fish
Whole Wheat

MANGANESE

Almonds
Walnuts
Peppermint
Parsley
Romaine
Dill
Liver
Chestnuts
Pignolia Nuts

SODIUM

Celery
Spinach
Swiss Chard
Romaine
Tomato
Radishes
Beets
Strawberries
Watercress
Pumpkin
Asparagus
Carrots
Leek
Dandelion
Rutabaga
Lettuce
Cabbage
Dill
Pomegranate
Butter
Okra
Cucumbers

SILICON

Rice
Strawberries
Pumpkin
Onions
Rhubarb
Parsnips
Spinach
Dandelion
Leek
Beets
Artichoke
Goat's Cheese
Whole Oats
Cabbage
Cucumbers
Apricots
Figs
Cherries

CHLORINE

Cow's Milk
Cottage Cheese
Eggplant
Coconut
Pineapple
Asparagus
Red Meat
Whole Wheat Bread
Sweet Potatoes
Sea Fish

IODINE

All Sea Foods
Salmon
Artichoke
Tomato
Natural Rice
Onions
Green Peas
Potato Skins
Pineapple
Grapes
Dulse
Kelp
Oysters
Turnips

SODIUM

Black Figs
Whey
Cabbage
Beets
Apples
Buttermilk
Avocado
Turnips
Pumpernickel
Banana
Roquefort Cheese
Goat's Cheese
Gizzards
Ox Joints
Gelatin
Eggs
Pistachio Nuts

10

How I Cured Myself of Hay Fever and Other Allergic Ailments

Hay fever is truly a dreadful affliction. I, for one, should know. I was miserably allergic to "ragweed" pollen, the most common hay fever allergy of all. It plagued me for about 20 years. I suffered with sneezing, wheezing, nose dripping, stuffiness, and watery eyes. It was so bad at times that I would have to sit up all night in a recliner, trying to sleep. It had me so exhausted that I often could barely catch my breath.

There is at least one consolation with all the suffering. Hay fever is seasonal. Ragweed is in full bloom in the late summer, during the months of August and September. When the pollen is in the air, it cannot be avoided. But once it is gone, you won't suffer until next year. Another respite for which I am thankful is that my hay fever lasted for only six weeks each year—some cases are known to last for two months and more.

There are various kinds of hay fever. The common ones involve weeds, flowers, feathers, hay, animal dander, house dust, and molds. Each year I struggled through the usual medical format of desensitization, injections, and drugs—mostly antihistamines and nosedrops. They brought some temporary relief, but they are known to have side effects and to be detrimental to your health. The drugs were so potent that they kept me in bed most of the time and made me lose my appetite and sense of balance.

A Startling Secret Discovery

It became apparent to me after a while that devitalization, nutritional deficiency, low resistance, faulty eating habits, excessive stress and strain, and insufficient rest were all at the bottom of this chronic, deep-seated disorder—and they gave it a chance to grow.

When you have suffered from such an affliction for about twenty years, you reach a point where you say to yourself, "I must do something about this invader that has been making my life miserable over the years."

For thousands of years doctors have been trying every known drug and treatment to conquer this horror, but no drug has ever completely cured the condition. I have never heard of a medical doctor who will tell you that hay fever can be cured.

A Difficult
Task in Store

Undaunted, and believing in miracles, I delved deeper into the matter. I felt that it would be best to continue with the drugs, tests, injections, antihistamines, and nosedrops for temporary relief until the natural methods—the traditional drugless healing therapies—could correct the cause.

Is a Change of Climate
the Answer to Hay Fever?

In the meantime, I remembered that I had read somewhere that Pikes Peak, highest of the Rocky Mountains (altitude 14,110 feet), was a haven for hay fever victims. It struck me as an interesting prospect for investigation, and so at the onset of the hay fever season, in the year 1947, my wife and I started out on an automobile trip from New York City to Manitou, Colorado, where we checked in at the Cliff House hotel, which is at the foot of Pikes Peak.

Ragweed Pollen Takes Over

We made a big mistake in not starting out for Pikes Peak a month earlier. Because we started our trip at the onset of the hay fever season, I had to visit different doctors along the way for the usual routine of drugs, etc. In addition, when we traveled through extensive areas of uncultivated land we often hit pockets of ragweed pollen.

We were so relieved when we finally arrived at the Cliff House hotel. After lunch, we took the cog train to the top of Pikes Peak. There we found unfortunate victims of various kinds of hay fever. They were sitting around in chairs scattered throughout the place, some on the outside, taking in the sun and fresh cold air. We found out that the scattered chairs on the inside were used as sleeping quarters by the guests, who would sleep sitting up in their outer clothing, sans pajamas, with the door to the outside closed at night.

Not My Cup of Tea

Noticeable through a glass enclosure was a refreshment room offering counter service. Just as my wife and I were about to go in for some refreshments, I was suddenly overcome with a choking sensation and shortness of breath. Nausea gripped me, and I got an uncontrollable nosebleed.

My wife, usually calm in an emergency, panicked and rushed me to the men's room and opened up the door for me. In I wobbled, trembling every step of the way. Once inside, I gave up everything I had eaten that day. I remained inside for a while, until my nerves were settled with a dose of ephedrine which I was lucky enough to have taken along with me. The whole thing was a complete surprise to me. I began to wonder, trying to put two and two together. I couldn't understand why all the other hay fever victims were getting satisfied relief, while I fell apart. The answer came soon enough. I managed to have a few words with a man who was trying to help me. We talked a few moments about allergies. His was "rose fever," and when I told him I suffered from ragweed pollen he told me, "Mister, you came to the wrong place." He explained that what will help me most is a low altitude and a warm dry climate, like Texas. I thanked him and hurried out.

Needless to say, my wife and I made a hurried retreat to the cog train and back to the Cliff House hotel where the warm fumes of a hot shower brought pleasing relief. We stayed on for a week and took the mineral baths in Manitou Springs, which were quite relaxing and exhilarating.

Warm, Dry Climate
the Best by Far

Since my wife's stepmother lived in Houston, Texas, we made Houston our next stop. The warm, dry, low-altitude climate was a step in the right direction. Though the hay fever season was not yet over, my physical well-being was greatly improved. My doctor in Houston reduced my usual format of drugs, etc., from once a day to only 3 times a week.

How and When
I Contracted Hay Fever

You sometimes wonder how you fall prey to an allergy. Someone or something must carry the blame. In looking back, I was able to trace the cause of my own allergy.

In my younger days, my father owned and operated a summer resort hotel in the Catskill Moutains, in an area close to a profusion of ragweed scattered throughout vast stretches of uncultivated land. I used to visit my father several times during the year, spending weekends at the hotel. I wondered if a combination of ragweed-polluted air and a period of low resistance on my part had caused the first symptoms of hay fever.

I put it to a test. On the onset of the hay fever season, I made it my business to spend a few weekends at the hotel. This sojourn was cut short when just three days later I made a hasty retreat back to the city—and to my doctor.

A series of allergy tests confirmed that I had a case of ragweed pollen hay fever.

A Step in the Right Direction

Many things began to dawn upon me. I began reading old and new medical books and medical journals pertaining to hay fever. I experimented with a few cures advocated by leading medical doctors, medical scientists, and researchers. Not one of these authorities came up with a complete cure. One leading doctor did, however, believe that nutrition could play an important part in the relief of hay fever. Although he did say "relief" and not "cure," it was a step in the right direction. This doctor expounded the fact that the modern diet is very bad because it is composed mostly of foods that have been altered by flavors, preservatives, and colorings, all of which are dangerous to health.

I would say that a person taking a proper diet, a natural diet—or what we call organic types of food—is in a better condition to fight against almost any common ailment.

Further researching revealed that such diseases as pellagra and scurvy went undiminished for years because the single vitamin remedy was overlooked. This struck a responsive chord in me. The question was what vitamin might it be that would bring about a complete recovery from hay fever.

An Encouraging Discovery

I chose the three efficacious vitamins A, E, and C for my experiment. I took the minimum requirements, one at a time, each day for two weeks. Vitamin C was the most effective. I began feeling much better. It was an encouraging sign. I hoped that I was on the road to a complete recovery.

I began taking the daily minimum requirement of vitamin C (300 mg.) until the onset of the hay fever season the following year. I was delightfully surprised to find that the usual symptoms were milder. But there was no sign of a complete recovery.

Increasing the
Dosage of Vitamin C

My medico was a great help by telling me that it was quite possible I wasn't taking enough vitamin C. He suggested that, six months before the start of the hay fever season, I take a total of 1,000 to 1,500 mg. of vitamin C each day, spread out in smaller doses throughout the day. Emphasizing the need for massive doses in my case, he suggested that I virtually saturate my body with vitamin C. He assured me that any excess is harmlessly excreted. That little I already knew. My doctor's suggestion reminded me of something I had found during my research in the medical literature: Massive doses of vitamin C play a very valuable clinical role in treating nasal allergy. Whether or not and to what extent the massive doses would work in my case was difficult to predict. All I could do was to hope for a cure-all.

My condition caused me to be confronted with a serious problem as to my personal life. Should I stay on in Houston and continue with the process of searching for a cure-all in a warm climate which allowed the minimization of drugs and injections? Or should I go back to home grounds in the north, carry on with further researching there, and be subjected again to intensive medical treatments until the natural methods could correct the cause?

It was a tough decision to make. I came to the conclusion that it was best not to change climates at that late stage in life, especially when my interests were ensconsed in the Northeast, where all my relatives, as well as long-time friends, were living. We returned home.

Here as fate would have it, my wife and I attended lectures by the late Helen Houston, a world renowned nutritionist, teacher, and health advisor. She described her regimen of inner cleansing, which became the basis of my nine-day inner cleansing and blood wash, the principal subject of this book. The purpose of Miss Houston's regimen was two-fold. First, to cleanse the blood and bring about the greatest possible elimination of accumulated poisonous waste, or toxins. These wastes have formed a lining around the intestinal wall within the body from childhood on, and, she said, they are the prime cause of disease. The second purpose was to supply the body with live, natural foods—foods rich in minerals and vitamins—to restore the much needed elements for cell rejuvenation.

Helen Houston was married to Dr. Douglas Urbanic, a chiropractor and nutritionist. My wife and I became students of her nightly classes, and after a year we had become so attached to her and her work that we helped her organize her nightly lectures, after which we would spend hours at a time in her hotel suite, talking about health.

A Suggestion for My Hay Fever

I lost no time in acquainting Helen Houston with the struggle to overcome my hay fever affliction. I related all my travels and everything that had been tried. She pointed out that if vitamin C had proved so effective, perhaps that Texas doctor knew what he was talking about when he recommended massive doses.

Miss Houston commented that the doctor should be commended for his broad-mindedness. As a rule, doctors have been satisfied with what they have been taught in their schools— only use drugs. It sounded to her like this doctor was becoming unorthodox.

In any event, she told me that I should try taking massive doses of vitamin C for my case of hay fever. It would not hurt me, and might do some good.

Before beginning this, however, she recommended that I undergo an internal cleansing to rid my body of poisonous waste. Then I should begin to eat foods high in vitamin C, such as carrots, celery, cabbage, apples, bananas, papayas, watermelon, beef liver, fresh fruit, and plenty of raw vegetables— the greener the better. I followed her advice, and also drank an average of from six to eight glassfuls of water daily, some fresh celery juice, and all the apple juice I could. I took a teaspoonful of wheat germ oil daily, and used honey as a sweetener in place of sugar. My main meals consisted of seafood three times a week, fowl twice a week, and broiled liver twice a week.

Abstinence from Faulty Foods

I abstained from condiments of all kinds, acid-forming foods, alcoholic beverages, carbonated drinks, salt, sugar, frozen foods, canned foods, pork, fried foods, starchy foods, preservatives, adulterated foods, processed foods, foods high in animal fats, sauces, gravies, coffee, tea, drugs in the form of laxatives and sedatives, saccharin, foods that contain white sugar, products made from white flour, synthetic sweeteners, and pills.

Our modern diet is so sickeningly altered, refined, and over processed.

The Happy Hour

When the hay fever season rolled around again, my mouth was agape when it became evident that all the symptoms of my disorder had vanished completely. The "small miracle" I had predicted right along and had been banking on was at last a reality. I can now go on a "hayride," should I so desire. To hay fever victims: "Have a happy August and September. It can be yours if you will follow my regimen religiously. Good luck!"

Of course, there were other natural measures I resorted to to bring about a cure, such as fasting twice a month, daily enemas and the traditional drugless healing systems and therapies.

Overcoming Allergic Ailments

At the time I was suffering from hay fever I was troubled with other allergic ailments, such as sinusitis, gastritis, chronic fatigue, bronchitis, high blood pressure, constipation, shortness of breath, acidosis, backache, and obesity. By employing the Nine-Day Inner Cleansing and Blood Wash and other required remedies and therapies, all allergy ailments should be overcome without much difficulty. It was hay fever and these common allergies that prompted me to embark on a course of therapeutic research so as to be able to cope with disease in the future without the use of drugs—and to help others who were suffering from disease. It was an exciting experience for me knowing that I would adjust my way of life and not repeat the same foolish mistakes that brought about my discomfort. My ill health was primarily due to dietetic errors and nutritional deficiency, which I now know to be at the bottom of every disease.

Chronic Fatigue

For chronic fatigue, I ate fish and other ocean food as often as possible. Ocean food is abundant in iodine and other minerals which medical research indicates sufferers of chronic fatigue need more than others. I swallowed one kelp tablet, rich in iodine, before each meal, and one before retiring.

Patients of chronic fatigue also need more iron. Iron builds healthy, red blood and deficiency in it is the most common cause of anemia, which is a serious form of extreme tiredness. Women have less iron than men. Eat a diet rich in iron.

Foods abundant in iron are: meat, liver, apricots, wheat germ, molasses, whole wheat bread, spinach, parsley, brewer's yeast, prunes, strawberries, tomatoes, cabbage, asparagus, watermelon, raisins, celery, carrots, grapes, radishes, cherries, cucumbers, black figs, and huckleberries. I recommend taking several tablets of desiccated liver several times a day. They are a good source of iron. Remember that vitamins E, C, and the B vitamins are a daily must.

Honey is a most effective remedy for chronic fatigue. Professional baseball players, football players, and basketball players are never without honey.

Gastritis

Gastritis usually comes from eating too much rich food or over-indulging in alcohol. To overcome it, take ample amounts of the B vitamins and calcium, get plenty of rest, and refrain from eating spicy, hard-to-digest foods. Papaya and peppermint are very helpful in soothing the entire digestive system.

Usually, gastritis will disappear completely if you refrain from rich foods and alcohol—especially beer—for a short period. I have know of instances where neglect in the treatment of gastritis has developed into mild ulcer attacks—in which event two ailments will have to be contended with, instead of one.

High Blood Pressure

The normal systolic blood pressure is between 100 and 140, and the lower diastolic pressure is between 60 and 90. A reading of 120/80 is considered normal. Those with diastolic pressure greater than 140 should be hospitalized.

A few tips on natural methods of lowering blood pressure: Garlic and onions are anti-hypertensive. Eat plenty of these vegetables daily. Indulge in regular exercise. Put in a one-hour workout at the gym or ride a bicycle five times a week. But if you are under treatment for high blood pressure, consult your doctor before taking exercise. People worry themselves sicker than they may be, in the belief that if they have slightly above-average blood pressure it may move toward higher pressure, heart failure or stroke, and death. Not true at all. In many cases, the blood pressure readings that are slightly above normal will either revert to normal at later rechecks or keep a safe, if slightly elevated, pressure for life. I know of a woman who has had higher blood pressure than average over 30 years and has never given any thought to it. Her doctor, a surgeon and general practitioner, was adamant in telling her not to worry about it until the pressure reached a reading of 120/80 or higher.

Dentists, as a rule, will not administer Pentothal Sodium (a temporary sleeping drug) to patients with high blood pressure. Yet, there are innumerable dentists who are not concerned with high blood pressure providing that the pressure reading is not much higher than 120/80.

It is indicated in medical circles that slightly above-average blood pressure is not as frightening as most people think.

How to Slim Down Without Dieting
or the Use of Drugs

High blood pressure is frequently associated with arteriosclerosis, heart failure, and/or heart attacks and hardening of the arteries. Since medical science has indicated for years that obesity, overeating, and eating the wrong kinds of foods are causes of high blood pressure, I recommend taking a teaspoonful of pure apple cider vinegar in a glass of water before each meal. Numerable cases of high blood pressure have been cured by blackstrap molasses and garlic, and I also recommend taking both of these "miracle" foods daily.

Bronchitis

Bronchitis may lead to emphysema if the respiratory tract is not kept clear of mucus. One way to keep it clean is to refrain from eating dairy foods and drinking cow's milk or homogenized milk. The juice of one lemon, taken three times daily, will help greatly in bringing up the mucus. Lemon is an excellent blood cleanser and helpful in obesity. It is a natural antiseptic agent, high in vitamin C—which you should take plenty of daily.

Sinusitis

Approximately 10 out of every 100 people who just have an ordinary cold believe they have sinusitis. A constant draining of mucus in the throat is actually the first sign of sinus trouble, accompanied by a clogged nose (known as postnasal drip). Vitamin A, zinc, potassium, calcium, and the elimination of cigarette smoking and alcohol will recreate healthy sinuses.

A Home Remedy for
Postnasal Drip

Using a mixture of one heaping teaspoonful of salt to a pint of warm water (shake well), lean your head forward over a basin of water and spray the mixture into each nostril five to ten times with a rubber eye syringe. Water will run into each nostril and out the other. Make sure that the nozzle of the syringe is all the way in each nostril. I have known this to be effective in opening up drainage and bringing up mucus.

Acidosis

Heartburn usually happens from twenty to sixty minutes after a meal, resulting as a rule from the kind of food you eat and drink. Condiments of all kinds and over-indulgence in coffee are contributing factors.

Acidosis will yield to peppermint, papaya, and pectin. Eat plenty of apples and drink all the pure apple juice you can. Vitamin C is very helpful. Complete fasting for a few days and a thorough rest generally help. Relax fully at mealtime, don't overeat, and for gratifying relief subsist mostly on dairy products.

Shortness of Breath

Shortness of breath is actually part and parcel of asthma. It is evident in medical circles that asthmatics have an excessive amount of potassium in their blood, and it is for this reason that I refrained from eating foods rich in potassium, such as tomatoes, kale, rhubarb, lettuce, turnips, celery, cabbage, rutabaga, swiss chard, cucumbers, watercress, beets, cauliflower, radishes, eggplant, lima beans, mushrooms, spinach, dill, limes, carrots, peaches. After a while, when it became evident that my shortness of breath was greatly improved, I began to partake of the vegetables I am most fond of, but not as often as I used to.

Marked increases in humidity are bad for asthmatics. Some doctors also believe that polluted air is bad for asthmatics. Most doctors, however, believe that the cause of asthma is largely emotional and hereditary. My shortness of breath was definitely hereditary. I can remember that my mother, God rest her soul, suffered from it interminably. It is known that chocolate is bad for asthmatics.

Backache

Backaches usually affect people who have reached middle age.

Here are some suggestions given by prominent orthorpedic surgeons to protect your back: Learn to sit in a straight-back chair, use a foot rest whenever you can, cross your knees when sitting; use a hard seat when driving; avoid lifting heavy objects; use a firm bed and firm mattress for sleeping; and take a hot shower for the sore area. Massages and chiropractic treatments are very effective.

Obesity

It is indicated in the medical profession that obesity is at the bottom of most diseases, and doctors find it very difficult to cope with them.

For complete recovery from obesity, I suggest: Refrain from all sugars—even fructose (natural sugar found in fruits)—beverages containing sugar, maple syrup, honey, molasses, prune juice, grape juice, all products made with sugar, all alcoholic beverages (especially beer), all products made with white flour, coffee, salt, highly salted foods, condiments of all kinds, smoked foods, fried foods, and pork.

Instead of three large meals daily, take frequent meals— several small ones. And don't gorge. Just nibble. Refrain from tidbits in between meals, and during TV programs. A good high protein breakfast is advisable. Include some lecithin in your diet. It helps to burn body fat. Vitamins such as E, C, A, and the B vitamins are absolutely necessary. Use plenty of them. Exercise can actually cut down the appetite. I suggest a 30 minute workout daily, preferably in the late afternoon. When you exercise, you eat less but enjoy it more. You will lose weight, and feel much more energetic. A balanced diet of nutritional foods is advisable.

11

The Seven-Day
Ever-Young
Diet

By using the word "diet," I do not mean a decrease in food for the purpose of losing weight. To diet is to control one's eating. It may signify, and generally does, a change in quality as much as in quantity. Control of diet results in weight control. It often prevents ill health, favoring the production of strength, vigor, and efficiency. On the other hand, unlicensed appetite and a diet that is not selective are responsible, in greater or lesser degree, for malnutrition or overweight, ulcer of the stomach, anemia, or other forms of ill-health.

Controlling Disease

I have spent considerable time in study and research in order to prepare a diet suitable in every way to the environmental and health requirements of the individual.

The wide range of carefully selected, tasty, nutritional foods contains practically all of the vitamins and minerals the body requires for the maintenance of normal blood pressure and normal weight, for controlling disease, and for the prolongation of youth. The diet has been so chosen as to keep it well balanced.

Our modern diet is so altered, refined, and over-processed that it lacks the balance of essential nutrients and enzymes needed to fight off disease.

Eat Your Way
Back to Health

The Seven-Day Ever-Young Diet is arranged in the form of menus that vary daily so that you will be eating foods that are high in vitamins and minerals and greatly effective in the healing and prevention of disease.

You may vary, to your individual desire, the kind of nutritious foods, fresh fruits, and juices that have been selected, providing that you do not have the same kind of foods and the same kind of juices too often. The Seven-Day Ever-Young Diet is truly a wonder diet. It is to be pursued every week during the year. Bear in mind that you have a variety of nutritional foods to choose from and that every menu will be different.

A list of these chosen foods, fruits, and juices follows:

VEGETABLES

Potatoes, sweet potatoes, rutabaga, cabbage, string beans, green peas, lima beans, cauliflower, beets, scallions, broccoli, Brussels sprouts, asparagus, carrots, celery, corn, spinach, swiss chard, kohlrabi, egg plant, onions, parsnip, turnip, dill, parsley, squash, pumpkin, artichoke, avocado, radishes, tomatoes, green peppers, lettuce, cucumbers, garlic.

FRUITS

Grapefruit, orange, apple, pear, banana, grape, prune, cantaloupe, watermelon, honey dew melon, casaba melon, peaches, strawberries, cherries, raspberries, blueberries, blackberries, nectarines, plums, coconut, pineapple, apricots, figs, dates, raisins.

JUICES

Orange, grapefruit, apple, pineapple, grape, prune, papaya, tomato, blackberry, cranberry, raspberry, apricot.

SEAFOOD

Flounder, mackerel, halibut, haddock, scrod, fillet of sole, bass, scallops, shrimp, cod, lobster, swordfish, salmon, salmon steak, crabs, tuna steak, tuna fish, frogs' legs, perch, trout, porgy, herring, sardines, whiting, weak fish, blue fish, water fish, shad, shad roe, pompano, smelts, red snapper, sturgeon, pike, mullet fish, lump fish, caviar, karp.

POULTRY

Chicken, turkey, duck, cornish hen, chicken livers.

MEATS

Lean steak, filet mignon, beef, roast beef, beef liver, lean lamb chops, roast lamb, pot roast, tongue.

SOUPS

Vegetable, potato, potato and onion, split pea, tomato, bean, mushroom, kasha, onion.

DESSERTS

Baked apple, apple sauce, nuts and raisins, stewed prunes, stewed figs, dates and nuts, fresh stewed peaches, brown rice with raisins and honey, stewed fresh pears, strawberries, melon, watermelon, blueberries, blackberries, banana with sour cream, health cookies, honey grahams, fresh fruit cup.

Recipes for Salads

GREEN SALAD

The salad consists of lettuce, cucumber, scallions, parsley, radishes, and beefsteak tomatoes. Dressing: sesame oil, minced garlic, paprika, apple cider vinegar, and some water. Shake well and serve cold.

COLE SLAW SALAD

Shred cabbage (remove outer leaves). Mix with dressing made of sesame oil, apple cider vinegar, minced garlic, paprika, and some water. Shake well, and serve cold.

WALDORF SALAD

Cut celery in pieces; peel and slice apples; sprinkle with pecans or walnuts; mix with French dressing. Shake well and serve cold.

AVOCADO SALAD

Avocado pared and sliced, grapefruit segments, orange segments. Mix with French dressing. Shake well and serve cold.

TOSSED SALAD

Lettuce, scallions, radishes, beefsteak tomatoes, water cress, cucumber, avocado, parsley, cabbage, carrot, green pepper—all cut into pieces. Mix with apple cider vinegar and sesame oil. Blend well and serve cold.

ROQUEFORT CHEESE SALAD

Put roquefort or blue cheese in a mixture of safflower oil, honey, apple cider vinegar, minced garlic, and paprika. Add some water. Shake well and serve cold.

Milk Sickness

I must dwell at some length on the habitual drinking of milk. It is indicated in medical circles that this is the third greatest destroyer of health. According to the Chairman of the Department of Medicine of the Harvard Medical School, Dr. Kirt Esselbacher, "Homogenized milk is one of the major causes of heart disease in the U.S."

Milk causes nasal congestion. It tends to generate excessive mucus in the intestines, sinus, and lungs. Excessive mucus generated by milk products is behind many respiratory ailments. It is an important factor causing postnasal drip and excessive phlegm in your throat.

One of the smartest things you can do is to cut milk from your diet. Replace it with skimmed milk or non-fat milk.

Pressurizing the Food You Eat

Most of the cooking done today destroys all the nutrients, because people do not know how to cook the natural way. The pressure cooker is a cooking utensil that possesses all the qualities conducive to better health. Health authorities agree that a pressure cooker provides the most modern, scientific method for retaining the nutrients in meats, vegetables, and fruits. The natural benefit to health cannot be over-emphasized.

A pressure cooker saves food flavors and color, saves cooking fuel, and prepares the tastiest foods.

Remember back when beans were cooked all day? Think of all the fuel consumed. You can prepare beans in the pressure cooker in about half an hour. How about clams in less than 5 minutes? Or shrimp in 2 minutes? When a recipe advises you to simmer meat 3 to 4 hours, the same operation can be done in a pressure cooker in only one hour—a saving of over 2 hours in gas or electricity and a saving of vitamins, minerals and taste.

Another advantage of pressure cookery is that you can cook several vegetables at one time. You can purchase a divider that separates the cooker into three sections.

Experiments in the chemistry laboratory of a highly rated university show that vegetables cooked in water for long periods lose the following minerals when the water is discarded: as much as fifty percent of the iron, forty-five percent of the phosphorus, and not less than thirty percent of the calcium. The water also contains a large portion of the vitamins and other nutrients.

Foods cooked the pressure cooker way are subjected to live steam at about 38 degrees Farenheit above the boiling point. Since a very small amount is used in cooking and the cooking is done in the shortest possible time, much of the health-giving qualities are retained. The juices contain much of the beneficial vitamins and minerals and should be used—never thrown away or wasted.

My wife and I have been using a pressure cooker for the past twenty-five years. This method of cooking not only has saved money on fuel but it has made food better tasting and more digestible.

Dr. Gene J. Riggins, director of the Clymer Health Clinic of Quakertown, Pennsylvania, has developed a "Power Packed Breakfast" which has a minimum of calories and a maximum of nutrition. It has proven itself to put "hustle in the muscle and vigor in the figure." Try it if you need a picker-upper at anytime. Here is the recipe:

> 1 to 2 glassfuls goat's milk or yogurt
> 1 to 2 raw fertile eggs
> 1 tablespoon wheat germ
> 1 tablespoon rice polishings
> 1 tablespoon brewer's yeast
> 1 tablespoon protein powder or skim milk
> 1 tablespoon lecithin
> 1 tablespoon liver powder
> 1 tablespoon bone meal
> 1 tablespoon unsulphured blackstrap molasses

Add cinnamon, nutmeg, or vanilla to flavor.

Blend in blender.

Ingredients should be kept refrigerated.

Supplies 350-400 calories and about 60 grams of protein.

I highly recommend this "power packed" breakfast once every week all year.

This Is for the Birds

I was taken aback by an article in the September, 1978 issue of *Moneysworth*. Here is an excerpt:

"Mount Sinai Hospital scientists say their tests show chicken soup is good for colds, and that it speeds the expulsion of germ-laden mucus from nasal passages, thus helping fight infection. They have labeled it 'efficacious upper respiratory tract infection therapy.' "

The reasoning of the Mount Sinai scientists is logically unsound. Chicken soup, especially the "home made" kind, is saturated with chicken fat which is decidedly detrimental to health in general—the same as all animal fat is harmful to your well-being. If anything, it will generate gobs of thick pasty mucus in the intestines, lungs, and throat, and very possibly cause bronchitis, postnasal drip, and other serious ailments. Under no circumstances whatsoever do I recommend chicken soup, even mother's kind.

The Seven-Day Ever-Young Diet contains a minimum of animal fat. On the diet, you will be eating fish three times a week, chicken twice a week, beef liver once a week, and lean meat once a week.

THE SEVEN-DAY EVER-YOUNG DIET

MONDAY

Breakfast

Before breakfast take a tablespoon of pure apple cider vinegar in a glass of warm water.

A glass of fresh orange juice; poached eggs on wholegrain toast, lightly buttered; Postum or herb tea with lemon juice and honey.

Before lunch have a glass of tomato juice.

Lunch

Sturgeon sandwich on pumpernickel bread; black olives; scallions; grapes; Postum or herb tea with lemon juice and honey.

Before dinner have a glass of apple juice.

Dinner

Baked fish garnished with minced garlic, lemon juice, and a thin cut of sweet butter; baked potato; spinach; avocado salad; apricots and nuts; Postum or herb tea with lemon juice and honey.

TUESDAY

Breakfast

Before breakfast take a tablespoon of pure apple cider vinegar in a glass of warm water.

A glass of fresh grapefruit juice; oatmeal with raisins and wheat germ; skimmed or non-fat milk; soft boiled egg; corn bread; Postum or herb tea with lemon juice and honey.

Before lunch have a glass of cranberry juice.

Lunch

Fresh vegetable soup; protein bread lightly buttered; carrot sticks; celery; raisins and sunflower seeds; Postum or herb tea with lemon juice and honey.

Before dinner have a glass of prune juice.

Dinner

Broiled beef liver and onions; broccoli; lima beans; bran muffins; green salad; stewed prunes and raisins; Postum or herb tea with lemon juice and honey.

WEDNESDAY

Breakfast

Before breakfast take a tablespoon of pure apple cider vinegar in a glass of warm water.

A glassful of pure apple juice; granola and wheat germ; skimmed or non-fat milk; hard boiled egg; wholegrain toast, lightly buttered; melon in season; Postum or herb tea with lemon juice and honey.

Before lunch have a glass of grape juice.

Lunch

Fresh Chinese vegetables (subgum) chop suey with brown rice, almonds, and kumquats; fortune cookies; Chinese tea.

Before dinner have a glass of carrot juice.

Dinner

Roast chicken with wheat germ stuffing; fresh asparagus; Waldorf salad; applesauce with raisins; health cookies; Postum or herb tea with lemon juice and honey.

THURSDAY

Breakfast

Before breakfast take a tablespoon of pure apple cider vinegar in a glass of warm water.

A glassful of cranberry juice; Ralston cereal with skimmed or non-fat milk; fresh apple; corn muffins; Postum or herb tea with lemon juice and honey.

Before lunch have a glass of papaya juice.

Lunch

Salmon sandwich with chopped onions that have been blended with apple cider vinegar; wholegrain bread; fresh pear; unsweetened grape juice.

Before dinner have a glass of raspberry juice.

Dinner

Baked fish garnished with minced garlic, lemon juice, a thin cut of sweet butter and paprika; sweet potato; carrots; tossed salad; baked apple; Postum or herb tea with lemon juice and honey.

FRIDAY

Breakfast

Before breakfast take a tablespoon of pure apple cider vinegar in a glass of warm water.

Half a grapefruit; soft boiled eggs; wholegrain toast, lightly buttered; banana; Postum or herb tea with lemon juice and honey.

Before lunch have a glass of buttermilk.

Lunch

Imported swiss cheese sandwich; whole wheat bread; apricots and nuts; Postum or herb tea with lemon juice and honey.

Before dinner have a glass of orange juice.

Dinner

Boiled chicken breast; string beans; corn

bread; cole slaw salad; stewed fresh pears; Postum or herb tea with lemon juice and honey.

SATURDAY

Breakfast

Before breakfast take a tablespoon of pure apple cider vinegar in warm water.

Unsweetened pineapple juice; Wheatena cereal with skimmed or non-fat milk; navel orange; bran muffins; Postum or herb tea with lemon juice and honey.

Before lunch have a glass of coconut juice.

Lunch

Nova Scotia sandwich on pumpernickel bread, lightly buttered; black olives; cole slaw garnished with apple cider vinegar; Postum or herb tea with lemon juice and honey.

Before dinner have a glass of celery juice.

Dinner

Baked fish garnished with minced garlic, lemon juice, paprika, and a thin slice of sweet butter; baked potato with chives and sour cream; cheese salad; dates and nuts; Postum or herb tea with lemon juice and honey.

SUNDAY

Breakfast

Before breakfast take a tablespoon of pure apple cider vinegar in warm water.

A glass of tomato juice; scrambled eggs prepared in corn oil; wholegrain toast, lightly buttered; fresh pear; Postum or herb tea with lemon juice and honey.

Before lunch have a glass of blackberry juice.

Lunch

Lima bean soup; tuna fish sandwich on wholegrain bread, lightly buttered, black olives; grapes; Postum or herb tea with lemon juice and honey.

Before dinner have a glass of spinach juice.

Dinner

Fillet mignon; baked potato; celery, carrot sticks; green salad; applesauce and raisins; Postum or herb tea with lemon juice and honey.

The Seven-Day Ever-Young Diet will give added strength to the body. Vim, vigor, and vitality will prevail at all times if this wonder diet is pursued religiously.

It is of special importance that a certain quantity of citrus fruits be taken daily, preferably by drinking their juices.

Drink 6 to 8 glasses of distilled water daily. No water with your meals.

Drink the juice of 3 lemons in water daily.

Take a raw egg yolk before lunch, and another in the mid-afternoon.

Drink all the apple juice you can daily.

Eat all the grapes you can daily.

Don't overeat. Sensible portions only.

Confine yourself to no more than three slices of bread daily.

Use corn oil in place of butter in preparing omelets, fried eggs, or scrambled eggs.

Avoid cream, meat stock, the skin of chicken, chicken soup, stews, gravies, or sauce. Eat the white meat of chicken only.

Take the minimum daily requirements of the major vitamins and minerals such as: vitamins E, C, A, B-Complex, B-6, B-12, kelp, bone meal, lecithin, brewer's yeast, dolomite, zinc, garlic, and potassium.

Never let a day go by without taking three teaspoons of un-sulphured blackstrap molasses.

Take a bowel flushing enema daily, and fast 2 days a month.

Take a teaspoon of apple cider vinegar, and one of honey at bedtime.

And last, but certainly not the least, don't forget to take the "Nine-Day Inner Cleansing and Blood Wash for Renewed Youthfulness and Health" in the late spring. It is your body's chief support and most powerful weapon against disease.

If you are seriously afflicted with a chronic disease, healing the body *first* by natural means is the chief discipline represented in the Nine-Day regimen. With the change to nutritionally controlled eating habits that you will experience on the Seven-Day Ever-Young Diet, you will be getting a new lease on life.

12

Powerful Weapons You Can Use to Overcome Major Diseases

The world around us is reverberating with new therapeutic and new world shaking theories about nutrition. Today doctors, medical scientists, researchers, nutritionists, and naturopaths discuss the need for improved nutrition. Medical writers have continued to report the latest developments in the use of vitamins and therapies for the treatment of disease. These developments have been taking place so rapidly that any one who has not made a special effort to keep abreast of the new developments will be amazed.

Vitamin pills were not available in my youth. In 1911 Dr. Casimir Funk discovered the first of the wonderful food factors to open the age of modern nutritional science. He called this "vitamin A." As other vitamin discoveries were made, they were called B, C, D, etc.

Action to Take Against
Degenerative Diseases

The degenerative diseases dealt with in this chapter are an outgrowth of undigested, uneliminated, unnatural food substances and foreign matter (poisonous wastes) that have accumulated and formed a lining around the intestinal wall from childhood on.

Disease is an effort of the body to eliminate the poisonous waste and toxins. The body must be cleansed and freed from such waste and foreign matter. In order to prevent and overcome disease, the body must be healed first. Medical doctors, as a rule, attack the disease first instead of trying to find out what the cause of disease is and heal the body.

The cleansing cannot be accomplished in a few days. Compensation must be made for the wrong committed against the body for a period of many years. The process of cleansing and healing the body must be systematic and general.

Action to
Overcome Pain

The beginning of every disease can be traced to the intestinal tract and to the food consumed. Knowing this to be a scientific fact, let us then intelligently search for the means that will help to eliminate the stored up waste and bring about a normal and natural function, thus restoring the body to its natural strength and radiant health. The more the body is free from obstruction, the more harmoniously and efficiently it will function.

Every pain that racks the flesh is the voice of Nature saying, unload, purify!

The course to pursue, in addition to the latest developments in the use of vitamins, supplements, and therapies is:

1. Detoxification of the body by the "Nine-Day Inner Cleansing and Blood Wash for Renewed Youthfulness and Health," to be employed six months apart the first year, and yearly thereafter. It will help to regulate high blood sugar and low blood sugar by cleansing the blood, will give the greatest source of relief from pain, and aid in the healing processes of disease, often bringing the body back to a normal state. Furthermore, it will help to avoid heart attacks, reduce the possibility of cancer of the rectum, which is increasing at an astonishing rate, and aid materially in overcoming obesity by slimming you down without dieting or the use of drugs—and it will keep you slim. It is nothing short of a simple and effective remedy with amazing self-restorative powers!

2. Taking Internal Baths (bowel flushing enemas) daily, will bring about "miraculous" changes in the healing processes of those suffering from disease—and those wishing to prevent disease. These fabulous internal baths will aid in reducing the possibility of cancer of the rectum, in warding off heart attacks, in detoxification, preventing constipation, and eliminating digested food before putrefaction sets in. Remember that incomplete bowel movements can be dangerous if allowed to stagnate. Gastro-intestinal upsets will vanish completely. In taking enemas, make sure there are no signs of appendicitis or other disorders. See Chapter 3 for more details.

3. Fasting one to two days a month will be very beneficial. It gives the body complete rest. As soon as you stop eating, elimination of poisonous wastes in the body begins to take place. The longer you go without food, the more waste matter is thrown into the blood stream, which carries it to the various organs of elimination. While this waste matter remains in the blood we become sick. Don't continue adding more waste to the already encumbered body with its ten to thirty pounds of stored up waste matter.

4. Eat your way back to health with foods that are high in vitamins and minerals and have a high chemical content. Don't dig your grave with a can opener.

Arthritis Is Far from Hopeless

Arthritis, a crippling disease, is an outgrowth of poisonous wastes (toxins) and foreign matter stored up and accumulated in the body over the years because of eating the wrong foods. While aspirin still remains the most widely effective drug in relief of arthritis because of its analgesic, or pain-killing effects, it is not without side effects. It is believed that over-dosage causes internal bleeding.

Doctors have recently recognized that a person who gets adequate amounts of vitamin C and other nutrients might very well never encounter arthritis in his or her life. Vitamin C is known to relieve some of the side effects of high-dosage aspirin treatment.

Vitamin E is also being used by many of the world's leading medical specialists in dealing with arthritis.

Honey is highly recommended by eminent nutritionists for the relief of pain in arthritis. Also, practically all doctors agree that exercise is one of the most important and beneficial therapies for this painful disorder.

Blackstrap molasses has been known to cure arthritis in its early stages.

Arthritic sufferers should avoid citrus fruits and juices. Celery and celery juice are known to be of great help. So is a daily tablespoon of wheat germ oil. Spicy foods and condiments of all kinds, starchy foods, tomatoes, tea, coffee and alcoholic beverages should be avoided. Eat only natural foods. Eat nothing sweet, except for fresh fruits.

Relief of the Strain
Put on the Body by Aspirin

Arthritics need more vitamin C. Doctors have recently recognized that when chronic arthritis patients were given adequate doses of vitamin C every day, not only would their pain lessen, but the body would also be relieved of the strain put on it by aspirin.

Spectacular Cures of Arthritis

Here are some case histories, spectacular in the rapidity of the cures:

Elaine B., 60 years old, had severe arthritis in her knees and hip joints. She was in a great deal of pain and was unable to walk without assistance. Finally, she tried blackstrap molasses. One week later, she could swing her legs and flex her knees—painlessly!

Mr. J, an elderly gentleman, was sorely afflicted with arthritis. Even with the support of walking sticks, he could barely hobble his way around. After four weeks of molasses therapy, he had improved so greatly that he threw away his sticks.

Drs. Thurman Bullock and Murray Carroll believe that at least 75 percent of arthritis conditions are caused by allergies to food, food additives, and chemical inhalants.

Heart Disease Controlled
in More Than One Way

It has come to be recognized in medical circles that sugar and salt are dangerous foods in heart disease. The first thing a doctor will tell you, if you have a heart condition, is to remove regular salt and white sugar from your diet.

You can reduce your risk of heart attack and stroke by moderate changes in living habits, says the American Heart Association. They suggest that you see your doctor regularly, avoid cigarettes and cigars, maintain normal weight and blood pressure, eat less saturated fats, and get regular exercise, based on your doctor's recommendations. Other leading causes of heart disease are excessive coffee intake, toxemia, malnutrition, and too little sleep.

A Powerful Weapon
Against Heart Disease

Of all the substances available to medical researchers, one of the most powerful and versatile is vitamin E. It is now being used by the world's leading specialists in dealing with heart and circulatory disorders.

The Shute physicians, of the Shute Foundation, London, Ontario, Canada, report they have evidence that vitamin E given in proper dosage prolongs the life of those who have had coronary attacks and so should always be considered by those who want to prevent such attacks.

Ingredients
That Strengthen the Heart

High blood pressure, according to some biochemists of the Dr. Schussler School, is frequently associated with arteriosclerosis, and like most afflictions that are curable at all, it is due to a deficiency of certain of the essential mineral salts. The most gratifying results have been obtained in many cases by the molasses treatment, plus the juice of one lemon a day. Molasses contains ingredients which are very strengthening to the heart muscles.

Case histories worthy of mention:

> **Several men who had been denied driver's licenses because of heart trouble were put on molasses therapy. After six weeks, they were cured and got their licenses.**

> **Robert D., a heart patient, was given a maximum of one week to live. His doctors had given up hope. But after taking blackstrap molasses for a period of time, he made a complete and miraculous recovery.**

> **A woman in her sixties had been afflicted with recurrent heart attacks for over three years. Treatments prescribed by her doctors gave her temporary relief but did not cure her condition. She took molasses a few weeks, and not only did her heart attacks cease, but she felt that her health as a whole had improved greatly.**

How to Decrease
the Need for Insulin

Diabetes is a degenerative disease and occurs more commonly in women than in men. The obvious cause is excessive use of sugar and starchy and fatty foods. Medical science indicates that for the most it is a disease of middle age and that there is often a predisposition for it.

Because there are few physical symptoms, the first indication is usually discovered by urinalysis and the presence of sugar in the urine. The most obvious symptom is a buildup of sugar in the blood and urine and consequent dehydration or dryness, resulting in thirst.

Insulin is definitely of great help in the relief of diabetes, but the need for it can be decreased by proper diet, keeping the body clean of poisonous wastes (toxins), and avoiding excessive weight. It is commonly known that many diabetics are overweight. However, I have found that reducing and keeping the weight normal or slightly sub-normal greatly improves the condition and results in needing less insulin. This in turn lessens the insulin's side-effects—hardening of the arteries, which may cause diabetics to be stricken at any time.

Foods Normalizing the
Blood Sugar in Insulin

The following are known to be of help in normalizing the blood sugar: egg yolks, garlic, brewer's yeast, whole cereals, dairy products, sauerkraut, green vegetables, all berries, cheese, lean meat, seafood, and grapes.

Good results may be achieved by going on a raw fruit and vegetable diet for a few days, several times a year. This should prove effective in diminishing the amount of sugar in the urine.

Dispense with saccharin or any other synthetic chemical sweeteners. I recommend "Fruit Sugar" (sparingly), which is obtainable at most health food stores.

A New Diet for Diabetics

In an article which appeared in *Prevention*, August, 1976, Dr. John M. Douglas explains that most people who followed his diet were able to reduce their requirement for insulin.

Dr. Douglas, a specialist in internal medicine with the Southern California Permanent Medicine Group, Los Angeles, has been helping his diabetic patients "keep the doctor away" by putting them on a raw-food diet. "I recommend raw foods such as vegetables, seeds, nuts, berries, melons, fruits, egg yolks, honey, oils, and goat's milk. Fruits, melons and honey were not to be eaten in large quantities, and nuts and salads were to be made the main part of the raw-food diet."

Most people who followed this diet were able to reduce their requirement for insulin, the drug diabetics need to help their body utilize the carbohydrates in their food. As Dr. Douglas said, "One patient had his insulin requirement reduced from 60 units a day to 15 units per day by dietary management alone, and another had his insulin requirement from 70 units per day to oral agents alone. Both of these changes were accomplished by increasing the percentage of raw food in their diets." In a more recent report, Dr. Douglas and a colleague, Dr. Irving Rasgon, chief of family practice, describe two diabetics who went on diets which were 90 to 100 percent raw. They were able to completely discontinue medication.

The rationale for prescribing the raw-food diet is based on Dr. Douglas' belief that early humans lived entirely on raw food, and that such a diet would be less stressful to the human system and less likely to produce diabetes than a cooked-food diet.

Dr. Douglas told *Prevention* that we all need the health benefits of raw food, whether or not we are diabetic.

We now find that the treatment of diabetics is incomplete without vitamin E. Dr. Evan Shute, prominent researcher of the Shute Clinic, has used vitamin E in treating some of the complications of diabetes. Dr. Shute prescribes high doses successfully even in extreme cases of blood vessel disease, where the patient has gangrene. Vitamin E given in proper dosage has made amputation unnecessary in some cases.

Any treatment with vitamin E that Dr. Shute prescribes for his diabetic patients is in addition to the insulin the patient normally takes. But some researchers have discovered that this does not always have to be the case. There are published reports that when the vitamin was administered in some cases, the need for insulin was eliminated.

Help for Emphysema Victims

Emphysema victims can breathe life back into their lungs.

In an article which appeared in *Prevention*, May, 1975, Michael Clark, associate editor, explains that the patient can't expel enough air to take in fresh air; victims work hard to breathe, even while asleep; the heart has to work overtime to pump blood through a damaged pair of lungs; and every day brings frequent coughing attacks.

Mr. Clark says there is no cure from this debilitating disease that turns a once-healthy individual into little more than an intelligent, wheezing vegetable, unable to do even the simplest of tasks, such as walking, without the most difficult effort. But there are two things that can help those suffering from the disease. One is a series of exercise. Although it can't be considered a cure, it allows emphysema sufferers to lead more or less normal lives by getting the lungs working again. On the other hand, research is beginning to show that better nutrition may prevent emphysema from developing in the first place.

For protection of your lungs, vitamins A and E are the best defenses against visible and invisible air pollutants that saturate our environment. New evidence has emerged which points out the protective role played by those vitamins in the face of contaminants involving the human lungs.

Graded bicycle exercise is an effective form of therapy for those suffering from emphysema.

Emphysema sufferers should abstain from smoking, alcoholic beverages, carbonated drinks, acid forming foods, condiments of all kinds, citrus fruits, food additives, salt, coffee, tea, white sugar products, white flour products, and homogenized milk.

Asthma Sufferers Find Relief

Asthma sufferers should overcome over-eating tendencies and eliminate and keep the body clean of toxins.

For a good sleep, take a tablespoon of corn oil at bedtime. Swallow one kelp tablet before each meal. Kelp is a natural supplement, grown in the ocean. It contains minerals, vitamins, and amino acids, particularly potassium and iodine. All of these help to keep the body calm and relieve nervous tension.

Incorrect breathing is a contributing cause of asthma. Do breathing exercises as often as possible, inhaling through the nose and exhaling through the mouth.

It now appears that vitamin A is playing an important part in the treatment of bronchial asthma.

Sufferers from severe forms of asthma should consult a "homeopathic" or biochemic practitioner, as few doctors are successful in dealing with this distressing complaint.

Regulating High Blood Pressure

High blood pressure is commonly known as a serious thing. Insurance companies, as a rule, will not issue a policy without first taking the applicant's blood pressure. Medical science has indicated for years that overeating is one of the causes of high blood pressure.

Action to Overcome High Blood Pressure

Excessive intake of meat, fried foods, pork, rich desserts, candy, sweets, cakes and cookies, fresh white bread, starches such as macaroni, spaghetti and the like, and thickened soups and gravy are considered to be an important dietary cause of high blood pressure. High blood pressure is frequently associated with arteriosclerosis, and if it is not brought under control, it may result in hardening of the arteries and ultimately heart failure and/or heart attack.

If you have high blood pressure, you don't know it. It often has no symptoms. It can be treated and controlled. The only way you will find out whether you have it is to be checked by your doctor at least twice a year. Persistent palpitation of the heart may be a warning, so heed such a warning and see your doctor.

Action to Heal Ulcers

Stomach ulcers are mostly attributed to the eating of present-day carbohydrates. To get effective relief from ulcers, you must abstain from any and all foods that contain refined sugar, and any and all products made from white flour. Omit from your daily diet acid forming fruits, fried foods, coffee, tea, carbonated drinks, alcoholic beverages, condiments of all kinds, and food additives. Refrain from smoking. Avoid salt and sugar as if they were poison. Use honey as a sweetener in place of sugar.

Eat only natural foods—and nothing sweet, except for fresh fruits and vegetables. Pure apple juice contains soothing properties and is most beneficial. Drink a glass or two at breakfast time, and throughout the day as your desire demands and your system allows.

According to practitioners of the Biochemic System of Medicine, ulcers do not occur unless there is a deficiency of certain mineral salts in the blood and tissues. As molasses, if taken over the requisite time, makes good that deficiency, it is not surprising to hear that gastric ulcers have yielded to that treatment.

A new hospital study shows that zinc helps heal—and possibly prevent—common stomach ulcers. The prescribed dosage of zinc is one tablet three times a day before meals.

Diet Conquers Psoriasis

Psoriasis, an eczema-like condition, is another dreadful affliction. You scratch yourself raw trying to shed the scaly patches that usually cover the entire body (but seldom the scalp). Turning from one doctor to another, from one salve to another, brings only temporary relief, and no cure seems to be in sight. Naturopathic physicians often prescribe a diet that should prove to be nutritionally effective in this skin disease. Or, as an alternative, they might advise a change of climate to Tuscon, Arizona where many psoriasis victims have found complete relief. My brother, age 78, has recovered from psoriasis by living in Tuscon for the past twenty years.

Since a skin disease is an attempt on the part of nature to rid the body of certain poisons, it would be wise to first get rid of that condition of the blood and tissues which is primarily responsible for the disorder, and then go on a prescribed diet of natural unadulterated foods, avoiding almost to exclusion carbohydrates, saturated fats, pork, fried foods, salt, white flour products, white sugar products, butter, condiments of all kinds, alcoholic beverages, carbonated beverages, and particularly all citrus fruits (which are known to cause an over-alkaline reaction).

High doses of vitamin A together with vitamin E are indicated to be extremely important to those afflicted with psoriasis.

Colitis Is Remediable

I have found that the most frequent cause of colitis is faulty eating. The wrong kind of food is certain to interfere with body chemistry and produce poisoning. Fortunately, it is remediable.

It is important to call attention to two other factors contributing to colitis which might be easily overlooked—that of over-eating, and that of being overweight. Colitis victims should refrain from stuffing themselves, and they should maintain a normal weight at all times.

In order to get relief, it is necessary to avoid almost to exclusion the use of condiments of all kinds, alcoholic beverages, soft drinks, adulterated foods, coffee, tea, citrus fruits or their juices, acid forming foods, fried foods, pork, vegetables with seeds in them, homogenized milk, white sugar foods, white flour products, and particularly roughage foods. Sufferers should eat no meat at all. Eat all the seafood you can and drink all the apple juice and papaya juice you can.

The carbohydrates are as much at fault as the meats. The sugars and sweets, rich desserts, heavy starches, and gravies are frequently the sources of fermentation. The natural sugars, such as occur in ripe fruits and honey, are less apt to cause this trouble.

The following foods and juices, as a rule, benefit colitis victims: dairy products like sour cream, cottage cheese, and yogurt (plain), avocado, watermelon when in season, goat's milk, coconut juice, and particularly buttermilk.

In the case of colitis, I recommend cooked vegetables in place of raw vegetables, since raw vegetables are harder to digest. They also contain a lot of roughage, which usually results in the inflammation of the mucous membrane of the colon.

13

My Lifestyle of Healthful Living— It Can Be Yours Too

I get up in the morning after nine hours of restful sleep, and I take a short nap in mid-afternoon.

Living in the city in a heavily trafficked area does not trouble me at all because I am never awakened by the deafening noise of the fire engines, ambulances, and automobile horns. God has endowed me with that gift— lucky me.

My wife tells me that if we were ever bombed during an invasion I'd go on sleeping. I am thoroughly relaxed when I get into bed and usually fall asleep the moment I am in the arms of Morpheus. Strange as it may seem, I believe I am capable of falling asleep standing up.

My wife, on the other hand, is highly attuned to noise. The buzzing of a weak bee in the far corner of the room will awaken her. Her sense of hearing is so acute she "can even hear the grass grow."

What I Eat Most

I've been maintaining my resistance with the following fresh fruits and vegetables, which I have especially chosen for their effectiveness in healing and warding off disease: cucumbers, asparagus, carrots, cabbage, apples, grapes. celery, pears, lettuce, tomatoes, peaches, coconuts, parsley, lemon, orange, grapefruit, onion, pineapple, spinach, banana, berries of all kinds, and melons when in season.

What I Don't Eat

I do not eat: processed foods, starches, adulterated foods, frozen foods, canned foods, carbonated drinks, homogenized milk, sweet cream, ice cream, pork, muscle meats, food high in animal fat, alcoholic beverages, salt, sugar, coffee, tea, rich desserts, sweets of all kinds, condiments of all kinds, sauces, gravies, saccharin, synthetic sweeteners, synthetic pills, drugs in the form of laxatives, sedatives, any and all foods that contain white sugar, and any and all products made from white flour.

Snacks Between Meals

For TV snacks and snacks between meals, I munch on black mission figs, pitted prunes, dates, apricots, raisins, nuts, and unsalted peanuts. Nuts are a high source of protein, particularly cashew nuts, which are complete in proteins. Brazil nuts are rich in calcium. Almonds are most nutritious. Pecans and walnuts are high in vitamin A, the healing medicine. Peanut butter, considered a legume, is rich in calcium and magnesium.

Processing destroys the foods we eat today. It causes a decline in health. The dangerous preservatives, bleaches, additives, dyes, and adulterates are slowly poisoning us.

Before we delve into the many facets of daily food consumption and therapies, we should know more about the major vitamins that sustain us, the proteins, the amino-acids, calcium, minerals, chlorophyll, and lecithin—all of which are likely barriers to serious diseases and conducive to healthful living.

The Mysterious Builders

The mysterious builders are the 16 minerals. Eleven of them are very essential, as they use the vitamins. Without them the vitamins cannot do their work. They are: calcium, chlorine, copper, iodine, iron, magnesium, manganese, sodium, potassium, phosphorus, and sulphur. They are the actual working catalysts—that is their super-function. When they are present in the body, the tissues are not torn down rapidly. They even help move the blood. Three of them, calcium, iron, and potassium, are essential for normal heart function. If the right proportions of these three are unbalanced for a long enough time, the heart stops.

Whole wheat, coconut, and egg yolk are all very special, because they contain these minerals. Without these minerals, the vitamins are useless in the body.

Calcium for Good Health

Most people are apt to suffer with a shortage of calcium. A loss of body energy is directly associated with a shortage of calcium. It has long been known that weakness of body and nerves, a below-par condition, or even serious disease can be a result of calcium starvation. It has been proven that a shortage of calcium in the diet causes a serious loss of potential body energy. About 25 per cent of the potential energy and 23 per cent of the protein value are wasted when calcium is lacking. This makes us realize just how dependent we are on calcium for good health. There is no substitute for it.

Protection from Infection

Vitamins in the food are the substances with which the endocrine glands are able to secrete. All ductless glands must have one or more of the vitamins in order to secrete their vital fluids, and if deprived of the vitamins, they will atrophy and cease to function.

The action of vitamin A is principally upon the epithelial surfaces, the skin and the mucus membranes, and in fact all of the lining surfaces from mouth to anus. Vitamin A protects us from infection at every point through which it might enter the body.

Stomach ulcers, infections of intestinal tract, colitis or ulcerations in any part of the intestinal tract all show a lack of protein, calcium, vitamin A, and vitamin C.

Vitamin A is definitely helpful in warding off the ravages of age, because in some fashion or another it protects the body from stone formation. Kidney stones and bladder and gall stones all show a deficiency of vitamin A. Research has shown that vitamin A increases the life span because of its influence on the glands. It helps to maintain alkalinity.

Vital to the Heart Action

Vitamin B is needed in the body to give tone to the muscles. It is vital to the heart action. It also contributes to the nutrition of the pituitary gland. It is essential to the welfare of the nervous system. Vitamin B is considered to be a 'pep' vitamin. Necessary in maintaining muscle tone in the intestines, it helps elimination.

Vitamin B deficiency is an important cause of hemorrhoids. Its lack can easily be responsible for the relaxation and congestion of veins, leading to the development of hemorrhoids. In severe B deficiency the blood vessels lose their tone and become enlarged and degenerated. Vitamin B enables the body to properly digest and convert the starches and sugars into energy.

The All Time Healer

Used in quantities, vitamin C (ascorbic acid) produces "impossible" cures. It is considered to be the all time healer. It keeps the arteries supple and young, and actually holds back the aging of the tissues. Degeneration occurs in the absence of vitamin C. It is essential for the proper formation and maintenance of bones and teeth, prevents pyorrhoea and promotes healthy gum tissues. Vitamin C hastens the healing of wounds, prevents infections, and protects capillaries against rupture.

Research by Dr. Emil Ginter, the eminent Czech biochemist, reveals that a lack of vitamin C often prevents the body from dispersing cholesterol build-up and may lead to two very widespread disorders, hardening of the arteries and gall stones.

Dr. W. J. McCormick, of Toronto, Canada, goes so far as to say that there is evidence that a lack of vitamin C might be one of the causes of cancer. We need more vitamin C as we get older. Studies have shown that it can prevent advancing age.

Vitamin D is essential for the utilization of calcium and phosphorus. Deficiency of D results in low serum calcium in the blood. Dietary calcium is not absorbed, and no calcium is made available in the serum to supply the tissues. We find it in few foods, so we must get it in sun light.

Vitamin F distributes calcium to the tissues. Lack of vitamin F causes dry skin. It is always found to be deficient in cases of anemia.

Vitamin G belongs to the B group. It is a precious food factor and has a profound effect upon the life processes as they relate to the aging of the tissues. It is essential to the breathing of the cells. This breathing, or cell respiration, is the method by which the living cell refreshes and cleanses itself. When the cell breathing is normal, the cells stay young. When the cell respiration is subdued, as it may be when Vitamin G is lacking, the cells shrink, grow old, and degenerate. This shows how important vitamins and minerals are. They must be supplied in adequate amounts before we can hope to rejuvenate.

Protecting the Body
Against Cancer

Vitamin E promotes the supply of magnesium and calcium to the tissues and helps to protect the body against cancer. It promotes the health of the sex organs.

Wonder of the Ages

Vitamin E is the latest vitamin recognized by the U.S. Government for its need in human nutrition. Of all the substances available to medical researchers, one of the most powerful is Vitamin E. I consider it to be the "wonder of the ages." It is being used by many of the leading medical specialists all over the world in dealing with heart and circulatory disorders, arthritis, diabetes, cancer, asthma, high blood pressure, emphysema, ulcers, anemia, colitis, varicose veins, sterility, mental retardation, and a host of other maladies.

The Hormone Generators

The next important food group to be considered in rebuilding of the body is the proteins. Liberal amounts of proteins step up the energy, increase the rate of metabolism, and keep the body at a high state of efficiency, of which one index is sexual activity.

The matter of choice in proteins is vitally important to you, as their amino-acids are linked up with hormones—the most powerful substances in the body. Meat, cheese, and eggs lead all other foods in furnishing all the amino-acids needed by the body.

You need an abundance of fruits and vegetables for vitamins and minerals, but their proteins are relatively inferior. In fact, a type of hunger-swelling, or water-logging of the tissues often develops due to a lack of certain amino-acids found only in perfect proteins.

Overcoming a Breakdown

The next important food substances are the lecithins. They promote the assimilation of albumen and the multiplication of cells, increase the red blood cells, and overcome nervous exhaustion. Pure lecithin is found in the brain and nerve cells. One cause of a nervous breakdown is lecithin hunger. Impoverished nerve tissue needs lecithin. Supply your body with plenty of it. It will increase energy, give strong recuperative powers, and bring back the memory. Without it, not even the life of a single cell would be possible.

Eat lecithin foods daily. Lecithin is found in egg yolk, salmon roe, calf liver, yeast, soy bean oil, and in the glands of animals. The egg yolk is the greatest source.

Another vitally important food element is chlorophyll, found in green leaves. This is the sun trap which stores the energy of the sun. Chlorophyll acts with the vitamins and minerals, the hormones and amino-acids, to produce the red pigment of blood cells. It has the power to protect the healthy cells against harmful bacteria by strengthening the cell structure.

Breathing and Exercise

Pure blood depends greatly upon the breathing power of the body. In its functioning, the brain uses up one half of all the oxygen that is absorbed by the lungs. Each nerve cell consumes four times as much oxygen as any muscle cell. The deeper you breathe, the more oxygen you inhale, and the purer your blood, the clearer your brain and the stronger the vital organs will be.

Five minutes of deep breathing will strengthen the body more than one hour of hard exercise. In connection with breathing, do your tensing exercise.

Good-bye to Cholesterol

A startling discovery! You won't have to go to the trouble anymore of looking into the history of every morsel of food before you put it into your mouth.

The medical profession, which for twenty years highly favored cholesterol, was stunned to learn from a Scandinavian study that cholesterol in food is innocent of any blame in causing high cholesterol levels in blood. The *New England Journal of Medicine* has now officially buried the concept of avoiding cholesterol in food. Many medical and scientific men have tried to show that prohibiting cholesterol will have no bearing on heart troubles.

A Startling Discovery

There is every indication in the medical profession that pyridoxine (vitamin B-6) plays an important part now in relieving three of the most pernicious diseases today—diabetes, hardening of the arteries, and chronic liver disease. It also acts as a mild diuretic. The minimum daily requirement of vitamin B-6 has not been established.

Digging Our Graves with Can Openers

Our modern diet is so altered, refined, and over-processed that it lacks the balance of essential nutrients and enzymes needed to fight disease. We are actually digging our graves with can openers.

Judging from present indications, there are approximately 400 different kinds of additives in our foods today, many of which have not as yet been tested by the Food and Drug Administration (FDA).

Since the present FDA regulations exempt food manufacturers from specifically listing all of the ingredients they add to certain food products, it seems evident that you cannot trust food labels. This is a serious situation since it may prove fatal to people who have dangerous allergies.

It is very important, for health's sake, to refrain from homogenized milk, cow's milk, and too much butter and cheddar cheese because they are mucous forming and bring on post-nasal drip and a host of other debilitating allergies. It takes five quarts of pasteurized milk to make one pound of cheddar cheese.

Burn Away That Fat

Upon rising, I take two teaspoons of pure apple cider vinegar in a glass of warm water—and two teaspoons before each meal. It will rid you of excess weight if you are obese and take inches off your waist, hips and thighs—and you will remain so. Cider vinegar has a tendency to burn away fat. It is nature's great health-promoter and safest cure for obesity. No other type of vinegar will produce the same therapeutic effects. It may justly be called a "natural wonder beverage." It is made from apples, which are perhaps the most health-giving fruits that exist. It promotes digestion and retards the onset of old age. Used as a gargle, it can cure a sore throat with astonishing rapidity. It cures or prevents the onset of many diseases.

I also take a tablespoon of unsulphured blackstrap molasses every night at bedtime. If people will not or cannot live on a well balanced diet, then the best thing to do is to consume as a daily habit at least one food which contains a large proportion of essentials to keep the blood and cells in a healthy condition. That food is none other than unsulphured blackstrap molasses. Blackstrap molasses can be obtained at any health food store or supermarket at a negligible cost. Among the numerous cases cured solely by molasses therapy are: growths of the uterus, growths of the breast, intestinal growths, growths of the tongue—all diagnosed as malignant. As for tumors, fibroid growths in various sites of the body have withered away without any other measures than that of taking molasses internally and using it in the form of poultices. It is exceedingly helpful in cases of arthritis, strokes, ulcers, eczema, psoriasis, high blood pressure, angina pectoris, weak heart, colitis, constipation, varicose veins, anemia, bladder troubles, gallstones, nerve cases, pregnancy, and "change of life." There is nothing like it for the prevention of the diseases mentioned above. Now you can see why I always take my quota of blackstrap molasses every day. I strongly recommend that you do the same thing. It's a must!

Don't ever eat because you have to eat. Eat only when you are hungry. There are times when I don't feel like eating anything and will skip a meal, taking fresh fruit juices instead. I call these lapses "short fasts." They give the gastric juices that are working all the time a chance to rest.

I eat all the grapes I can when in season. They assist the body in burning some of its stored fat, at the same time keeping the sugar from falling too low. They are good blood and body builders. Grapes are recommended for diabetics or people allergic to diarrhea.

I drink all the apple juice I can. "An apple a day keeps the doctor away" is no empty slogan, for apples contain some important chemical ingredients. They render the urine normal, thus counteracting an urge to urinate too frequently. They affect the blood, making it of the right consistency, regulate menstruation, cure and prevent obesity, and promote digestion. They act as a preventive in so many of our common ailments.

The Major Preventives of Disease

The following are the major type of vitamins and supplements I take every day to ward off disease: Vitamins E, C, A, B-6, B-12, B-Complex, kelp, bone meal, lecithin, dolomite, zinc, and brewer's yeast. I take double the daily minimum requirement of vitamin E, vitamin C, vitamin A, lecithin and brewer's yeast.

An Amazing Powerhouse
of Nutrition

One of nature's most fantastic sources of nutritional benefits is brewer's yeast. It is naturally packed with food energy and B vitamins. For thousands of years, yeast has been used in baking, wine-making and brewing, and now it has been discovered to be a valuable food on its own. Each tiny brewer's yeast cell is rich in protein (just like human body cells) and contains an amazing powerhouse of natural vitamins, minerals, carbohydrates, enzymes, and *all* the essential amino acids! It is regarded as one of nature's most complete and "perfect" foods.

I use whole grain bread, no more than 3 slices a day, plain or toasted.

I drink two glasses of buttermilk daily.

I drink 6 glasses of distilled water daily.

I have with my evening meal a large green salad with dressing made of sesame oil, apple cider vinegar, paprika, honey and some water, served cold.

I drink the juice of one lemon in water daily, usually in the late afternoon. It is a high source of vitamin C, an excellent blood cleanser, and a natural antiseptic. Most importantly, it will help in the elimination of mucus.

I eat seafood three times a week, fowl twice a week, beef liver once a week, and lean meat once a week.

Controlling Disease with
the Ever-Young Diet

I take the Seven-Day Ever-Young Diet in the fall, and the alternate Seven-day diet in the late spring. See Chapter 11. The wide range of carefully selected nutritional foods contains practically all of the vitamins and minerals the body requires to ward off disease. The diet has been so chosen as to keep it well balanced. It contains a "power-packed" breakfast to be taken once a week.

The "Nine-Day Inner Cleansing and Blood Wash for renewed Youthfulness and Health," which I take yearly, has warded off common ailments and the most pernicious diseases. It has kept me in the best of health throughout the years.

A

A, vitamin:
. acne, 104-105
. aging, 97, 98
. albuminuria, 98
. asthma, 195
. bowel function, 98
. bronchitis, 106
. cancer, 100-103
. carotene, 98, 99
. cod liver oil, 100
. colds, 98, 99, 100, 104
. colitis, 98
. cystitis, 98
. discovery, 85, 103-104, 185
. dropsy, 98
. epithelial surfaces, 97, 98, 99
. eyes, 97, 100, 103
. filterable virus, 99
. gastritis, 98
. glands, 97, 98
. growth, 97
. infection, 97-99, 101, 104, 204
. influenza, 99, 100
. intestinal tract, 98
. jaundice, 99
. kidney function, 98
. lack of appetite, 98

A, Vitamin (*cont.*)
. lactation, 104
. liver function, 98
. lungs, 194
. mastoid, 99
. natural sources, 97, 99, 105
. nephritis, 98
. psoriasis, 105-106, 198
. pus germs, 99, 104
. reproduction, 104
. results of deficiency, 102-103, 103-104
. rickets, 100
. sinuses, 99, 103
. stone formation, 97, 98
. storing, 104
. stress, 100
. tonsils, 99, 103
. ulcers, 98, 100
. vitamin E cooperates, 83
Abortion, recovery, 85
Abrahamson, E.M., 128
Acidosis, 167
Acne, 24, 104, 105
Acute thrombosis, 84
Additives, chemical, 128-130
Aging, 88, 97, 98, 206
Airola, Paavo, 128
Albuminuria, 98
Alcoholism, 127

217